ONCE A MONTH

————————— 🐌 —————————

"This book is written with the aim of spreading the news that the once-a-month miseries of countless women can be, and are being, successfully treated and relieved. It is also written to help men understand and appreciate the menstrual problems of women, and become partners in helping them through their difficult days. That you are reading this book brings hope that the aim will be achieved."

—From the Book

"ONCE A MONTH is the single most important book I have ever read. It certainly saved my sanity and quite possibly my life. You can't know how grateful I am to you—and the gratitude is profoundly shared by my husband and our son."

—M.T.I., Waynesburg, Pa.

About the Author

———— ❧ ————

Katharina Dalton was born in England in 1916. Her early training was as a chiropodist at the London Foot Hospital, where she wrote *Essentials of Chiropody*, now a basic textbook. Widowed with one child during the war, she started medical training at the Royal Free Hospital, worked in the evenings, remarried, and had three more children. In 1948 she qualified as an M.D. and entered general practice where, during the first two months, she identified and successfully treated six women suffering from premenstrually related asthma, epilepsy, and migraine. For 32 years she has continued researching premenstrual syndrome in her extensive practice. This interest resulted in 1953 in the first paper in British medical literature on premenstrual syndrome, written in collaboration with Dr. Raymond Greene. In 1954 her work with premenstrual syndrome patients at University College Hospital, London, led to her establishing there the world's first and oldest premenstrual syndrome clinic, which she still maintains and where, in conjunction with her Harley Street practice, she continues her studies into premenstrual syndrome and related illnesses.

Dr. Dalton is now an acknowledged authority on the part played by menstrual dysfunctions in confused and criminal behavior, accidents, drug abuse, and morbidity. Her work on premenstrual syndrome and its treatment with progesterone therapy is applied in factories, schools, prisons, shops, and hospitals, and she has received widespread recognition for her research. She has been awarded the Charles Oliver Hawthorne BMA prize for outstanding research in general practice on three occasions, and has also received the Upjohn Fellowship, the

About the Author (continued)

Charlotte Brown prize and the Cullen prize from the Royal Free Hospital, and the British Migraine Association prize from the Royal College of General Practioners, of which she was a founding member. In 1971 she became the first woman President of the General Practice section of the Royal Society of Medicine. In 1980 she was the expert witness in two cases of murder in which premenstrual syndrome was first accepted as a factor causing diminished responsibility, thus making legal history in Britain. She was awarded the Fellowship of the Royal College of General Practitioners in 1982.

Her books and publications have been translated into 12 languages, and include *The Premenstrual Syndrome* (1964), *The Menstrual Cycle* (1970), *The Premenstrual Syndrome and Progesterone Therapy* (1977, 2d ed. 1984), *Depression after Childbirth* (1980, 2d ed. 1990), *Premenstrual Syndrome Illustrated* (1990), and *Premenstrual Syndrome Goes to Court* (1990). She has lectured extensively to both medical and lay audiences all over the world and has made numerous radio and TV appearances in Europe and the United States.

Dr. Dalton is married to a Unitarian minister and has four children and five grandchildren.

ONCE A MONTH

The *Original* Premenstrual Syndrome Handbook

———————— ❧ ————————

KATHARINA DALTON, M.D.

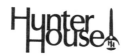

Library of Congress Cataloging-in-Publication Data:

Dalton, Katharina, 1916-
> Once a Month : the original premenstrual syndrome handbook / Katharina Dalton. — 4th rev. ed.
>> p. cm.
> ISBN 0-89793-071-1 : $9.95
> 1. Premenstrual syndrome. 2. Menstruation disorders. I. Title.
RG165.D34 1990
618.1'72—dc20   90-4543
                                                                      CIP

Cover design by Tamra Goris
Book design by Qalagraphia
Copy editing by Connie Salveta, Corrine Sahli, and K. S. Rana
Production manager: Paul J. Frindt
Set in 11/13 Goudy Old Style by 847 Communications, Claremont CA
Printed and bound by Delta Lithograph Co., Valencia, CA
Manufactured in the United States of America

9 8 7 6 5 4 3 2 1   4th edition

Contents

List of Figures ix

Preface to the First Edition xi

Preface to the Second Edition xii

Preface to the Third Edition xiii

Preface to the Fourth Edition xvi

Introduction 1

1   The Curse of Eve 5

2   Mood Swings 16

3   Clearing the Confusion 21

4   Premenstrual Tension 35

5   Waterlogged 47

6   Monthly Headaches 54

7   Recurrent Problems 63

8   Pain and Periods 73

9   Awkward Adolescent 81

10   Marriage 90

11   Advice to Men 100

12   Mother 107

13   The World's Workers 115

14   Women at Leisure 121

15   Premenstrual Syndrome Goes to Court 128

16   The Hormonal Control 135

17   What Goes Wrong? 153

18   After A Hysterectomy or Oophorectomy 162

19   Menopausal Miseries 169

20   Helping Yourself 185

21   What Can the Doctor Do? 194

22   A Fairer Future 216

     Glossary 223

     Other Publications by the Author 227

     Resources: PMS Clinics and Support Groups in
        the U.S.A. 235

     INDEX 245

List of Figures

1   Menstrual hormone variations during the menstrual cycle 13

2   Male hormone levels during a month 13

3   A simple menstrual chart 25

4   Menstrual charts diagnostic of premenstrual syndrome 26

5   Menstrual chart with unrelated symptoms 27

6   Chart of adolescent girl with cyclical symptoms before the start of menstruation 28

7   SHBG-binding capacity in 50 patients with severe premenstrual syndrome compared with 50 symptom-free controls 30

8   Effect of progesterone on SHBG levels 31

9   Variation in schoolgirls' weekly grades with menstruation 42

10   Fluctuations during the menstrual cycle in weight, blood pressure, and pressure in the eye of a sufferer of premenstrual syndrome 48

11   935 migraine attacks in relation to the menstrual cycle 55

12   Headaches in relation to menstruation 56

13   Sites of greatest pain in menstrual headaches 57

14   An attack form useful for isolating trigger factors in migraine 59

15   Common symptoms of premenstrual syndrome 66

16   Charts of two patients with premenstrual epilepsy . . 67

17   Site of pain in spasmodic dysmenorrhea 76

18   The position of organs around the womb 79

19   Female development at puberty 82

20   Position of the menstrual clock 138

21   Diagram of controlling centers in the
      hypothalamus 138

22   Menstrual hormonal pathways 140

23   Temperature charts taken through the menstrual
      cycle 142

24   Timing of ovulation with different lengths of
      cycles 143

25   Levels of progesterone during the menstrual cycle
      and pregnancy 148

26   Effect of food on blood sugar levels 150

27   Effect of food on blood sugar levels in women
      with premenstrual syndrome 151

28   Arbitrary levels of progesterone and estrogen 156

29   Hormonal pathways in menstruating and
      menopausal women 171

30   Need for estrogen therapy at menopause 173

31   Relation between the age of menarche and
      menopause 175

32   Signs of estrogen deficiency at menopause 179

33   Relation between armspan and height   181

34   Effect of progestogen on the blood level of
      progesterone 209

35   Symptoms of Vitamin B-6 overdose 213

Preface to
First Edition

ब

This book is dedicated to the thousands of women who have confided in me the most personal and intimate details of their lives and from whom I have learned so much.

I am deeply grateful for the help received from all my family. To Drs. Maureen and Michael Dalton who have been my most severe critics; to Mrs. Anita Dalton and Mrs. Wendy Holton who have patiently typed, corrected, and retyped the manuscript before it was ready for submission to the publishers; to my niece Mrs. Sherryl Machray for the artwork; to Mrs. Sharlynn Orr who has kindly adapted my work for America; and most of all to my long-suffering husband, Rev. Tom Dalton, for his invaluable ghost-writing of the entire book.

Finally, my acknowledgment to David Duff and Tandem Press for the excerpt from *Albert & Victoria*, and the Journal of the Royal College of General Practitioners for their permission to reproduce Figure 11.

Katharina Dalton
1978

Preface to
Second Edition

—————————— ❧ ——————————

In 1954, speaking to the General Practice Section of the Royal
Society of Medicine, I ended my paper with the words:

> "The cost of progesterone therapy is high, but when this is
> weighed against the price in terms of human misery, suffer-
> ing and injustice, it is seen as a justifiable expense opening
> up a new vista of Medicine."

That vista is still opening up and during the last few years
considerable progress has been made in the appreciation and
understanding of menstrual problems and their treatment by the
caring professions and also by the general public.

At the symposium on Premenstrual Syndrome at the International Congress of Psychosomatic Obstetrics and Gynecology
held in Berlin in September 1980, it was agreed that premenstrual syndrome was a hormonal disease, therefore it was more
suited for study by international meetings of endocrinologists
rather than by psychologists. Of course there will always be
those who disagree and suggest other approaches, which is as it
should be, provided they are talking about the same diagnosed
disease and have tried the same treatments, comparing them
with other treatments to find the most successful.

New issues have emerged, such as the legal implications
and the feminist movement. Premenstrual syndrome should not
be a feminist issue. It is a hormonal disease, which deserves sympathy and understanding and requires to be diagnosed and treated.

This edition has been widely revised in light of the findings of the past four years. It is as up-to-date as possible, in the
hope that the disease will be more commonly recognized, correctly diagnosed, and properly treated.

Katharina Dalton
London, 1983

Preface to the Third Edition

—————— ❧ ——————

The need for a third edition is a clear indicator that the demand for authentic information on premenstrual syndrome is in no way slowing down. Nor, regrettably, are the torrents of misinformation, false information, mythical treatments, and armchair theories. Indeed, it is these outpourings that are creating the confusion, not merely among the unfortunate sufferers of premenstrual syndrome, but also among the public, social workers, and other health professionals. This adds a greater urgency to the need to provide a third edition based on the experience accumulated during more than 38 years of continual work with this pernicious disease.

There have been considerable advances in our knowledge of a woman's reproductive processes since this book was first written in 1977. These include the realization that each woman's menstrual cycle follows her own individual pattern, which can vary considerably from woman to woman and yet remain normal; an appreciation that hormones are multifunctional; and an understanding of their behavior, their transport through the body, and their interactions within the target cell. Of particular importance are the recognition of progesterone receptors in the midbrain and the value of an estimation of the binding capacity of sex hormone binding globulin (SHBG). But there is still much ignorance and many questions that need to be answered. New knowledge on the subject is eagerly awaited to help in solving some of the remaining mysteries.

Meanwhile, there remains a need for self-help groups to assist women in making the connection between their symptoms and menstruation; to instruct in menstrual charting; to teach the essential dietary rule of eating some starchy food every three hours; and to point the sufferer toward sympathetic medical practitioners ready to prescribe effective treatment to eliminate monthly problems. Groups can agitate for the inclusion of premenstrual syndrome in the medical curriculum at both undergraduate and postgraduate levels, ensure that adequate funds are available for research and clinical trials, and educate society to recognize that premenstrual syndrome is a hormonal and not a psychological disorder. In 1986 American women showed their strength by overturning the American Psychiatric Association's desire to see premenstrual syndrome labeled as a mental disease.

In this edition a new chapter, "Clearing the Confusion," has been added to help readers verify the authenticity of what they read and hear about premenstrual syndrome. It also explains the difficulty of trying to diagnose premenstrual syndrome correctly, using conventional methods of diagnosis. There is new information in almost every chapter, although some are more altered than others.

"Nature knows no pause in progress and development and attaches her curse on all inaction." Both aspects of Goethe's nineteenth-century saying are to be found in the story of premenstrual syndrome. The ongoing progress and development is to be found in my many writings from 1953 to the present, and is reflected in the never-ending stream of women referred daily for diagnosis and treatment. The other side, Nature's curse, is experienced by those countless women whose premenstrual sufferings continue because of the unwillingness of practitioners to use effective progesterone treatment until its success has been proven in double-blind placebo controlled trials. To some that may sound a reasonable excuse for inaction, but let us take a lesson from history. Scurvy was the major cause of mortality and morbidity among sailors on long sea voyages, until the sixteenth century, when the Dutch discovered the value of a diet containing citrus fruits with which to combat scurvy. Nevertheless, it was not until 1932 that vitamin C (ascorbic acid) was identified as the curative agent in the fruit. In those earlier years no one felt the need to wait three centuries until science found the evidence—"the proof of the pudding lay in the eating," so to speak—and consequently many thousands of lives were saved from the ravages of scurvy. Today, the women suffering from premenstrual syndrome who have been properly treated with progesterone know how very effective it is. Do the others have to wait 300 years until we know the exact mechanism of its action, or are they deserving of treatment now?

During the preparation of this third edition that question has been in the forefront of my mind, alongside another one: how can I encourage my colleagues to learn the necessary new skills to enable them to correctly diagnose and properly treat premenstrual syndrome? This book has been written in the firm belief that all who read it with an open and unprejudiced mind will be able to learn a great deal about premenstrual syndrome and the reason for its treatment with progesterone. They will also appreciate that it is a very real disease that can have extremely serious consequences for some of its sufferers, but a disease that has responded magnificently to progesterone treatment ever since this was first used in 1948.

It now remains for me to continue with my work of healing and to express my gratitude to all those patients who have taught me so much; also to the many colleagues who have contributed to the development and increase of my understanding of endocrine involvement in the disease, particularly my daughter, Dr. Maureen Dalton. These thanks would not be complete without an acknowledgment of the invaluable contribution of my hardworking staff, especially Wendy Holton and Jane Rogers. As always, your thanks and mine must go to my husband, the Rev. Tom Dalton, for all his support and untiring determination to maintain a high standard of readability for your enlightenment and pleasure. Finally, my acknowledgment to William Heinemann Medical Books Ltd. for permission to reproduce Figures 7 and 8 from my book *Premenstrual Syndrome and Progesterone Therapy*.

Katharina Dalton
London, 1987

Preface to the Fourth Edition

————————— 🐌 —————————

This new edition is not only evidence of the success of this popular book on premenstrual syndrome, it is also an indication of the importance and value of the information it provides for recognizing, diagnosing, and understanding this distinctive woman's disease.

The high standards established in this book reflect the knowledge gained in over 40 years of daily consultations, diagnosis, and treatment of a wide range of PMS patients from all corners of the earth, each with her differing severities, presentations, and need for personalized treatment. This knowledge is enhanced by a continual scrutiny of worldwide medical and scientific research on the subject, especially of the animal biologists and their work on progesterone receptors. Many of these people see their work as being of purely scientific interest, but that is not so. Their findings are of real importance to us today, providing as they do a greater understanding of the little-known, but vital, functions of progesterone, receptor sites, and progesterone receptors. A full understanding of their work enables the PMS doctor to make a larger contribution to the good health of the patient and all members of her family.

"The art of medicine is valuable to us because it is conducive to health, not because of its scientific interest." So wrote Cicero in the pre-Christian era, and this is, of course, the justification for this new, carefully revised and up-to-date edition. Among those especially deserving of my thanks for their help and support are the many sparring partners who, over meals or late into the night, have discussed and dissected new findings, theories, and ideas. Foremost among them have been my family, with the Reverend Tom trying to clarify my thoughts and understand the arguments propounded by Drs. Michael and

Maureen Dalton, and Mrs. Wendy Holton, as well as Dr. Niall MacKenzie and Dr. Ian Simpson, not forgetting Dr. Glenn Bair in Topeka and Dr. Mary Cortner in Kansas City. My thanks go to them all, and to those unknown scientific workers who have given us so much food for thought.

Katharina Dalton
London, May 1990

Introduction

———— ❧ ————

Once a month, with monotonous regularity, chaos is inflicted on American homes as premenstrual tension and other menstrual problems recur time and time again with demoralizing repetition. Wonderfully happy and often long-term marriages and partnerships break up under the strain because one partner is an unpredictable, irrational, and often violent woman suffering from premenstrual syndrome. In such a situation the man may decide that there is no future for the relationship, and leave. He may feel bound to stand by his wife and their children, in which case he will have to face up to a hard time learning to live with all kinds of disconcerting situations.

It is important that men *do* learn that the relationship is not doomed, however, for once the woman's premenstrual syndrome has been recognized and correctly diagnosed, it can be successfully treated. This book explains how these premenstrual problems can be completely relieved with the proper treatment, just as the pains of childbirth are today universally treated with pain-relievers and anesthetics.

It has also been written to help men understand the cause of these capricious and temperamental changes in women, so that the image of woman as uncertain, fickle, changeable, moody, and hard to please may go, to be replaced with the recognition that all these features can be understood in terms of the ever-changing ebb and flow of her menstrual hormones and the hormonal changes they cause within her body's cells.

It was as long ago as 1948 that I came across my first case of premenstrual asthma, which responded successfully to treatment with progesterone. Before a month had passed, a further case of asthma, two of epilepsy, and one of migraine had been found, all related to menstruation. However, for premenstrual syndrome to be properly appreciated, it must be recognized in its full variety. Following a television documentary on the subject which showed four situations—an alcoholic, a baby-batterer, a husband beater, and a neurotic—the hospital's mailbox was filled with letters that suggested the program had been an eye-opener to many viewers. The letters contained such comments as:

"It was such a relief to know that so many other women experience the very real and deep feelings of anger, hatred, and depression that I feel in the days before my period."

"I'm just like that woman."

"I never told anyone because I thought they would never believe me."

It is hoped that this book will open many more eyes. It is estimated that there are in America today over 5½ million women with incapacitating monthly problems that can and should be eased.

The first step is to bring the subject out into the open, not to sweep it under the carpet. Menstruation should be a subject that can be discussed as openly as sex: anywhere, by anybody, not only in the bedroom or doctor's office. We still suffer from the utterly Victorian attitude in which heroines in novels never menstruate. Since the first edition of this book in 1978 there has been a most productive opening up of the subject. Indeed, PMS is now the widely recognized abbreviation of premenstrual syndrome and is a favorite topic for many women's journals, yet even today it is not routinely accepted as a hormone disorder. If women themselves do not associate the changes in their body and psyche with the changes in menstrual hormones, how can one hope that men will be able to understand them? After all, men don't even experience these changes. There *must* be a general recognition of the physical and psychological changes in a woman, which occur like a flash of lightning before menstruation, and which are not due to personality inadequacies.

While fatalities from premenstrual syndrome or period pains are rare and the suffering is short-lived, ending with menstruation, nevertheless the suffering, unhappiness, and social consequences of PMS are without limitation.

One gynecologist ranks premenstrual syndrome as the most common cause of marital breakdown. In a survey in England, 75% of a sample of 521 women complained of at least one premenstrual symptom. Also in England the attempted suicide rate shows that there is a sevenfold increase in the second half of the menstrual cycle compared with the pre-ovulatory half. Shoplifting is 30 times commoner in the second half of the cycle. As long ago as 1977 it was found that of 132 women who were currently under the care of the Premenstrual Syndrome Clinic at University College Hospital, London, 37% had a previous mental hospital admission; 34% had attempted suicide or homicide; 9% had alcoholic bouts; 6% were referred because of actual child abuse, and a further 4% sought treatment because of a fear of their injuries to their children becoming public knowledge; 6% had a history of criminal behavior, such as smashing the windows of the Social Services headquarters and assaulting police or neighbors; 7% had premenstrual epilepsy; and 5% had premenstrual asthma.

These are not trivialities, but are matters of vital concern to the patient, her family, society, and maybe even the nation. This is shown in the following extract from *Albert & Victoria*, David Duff's book on the married life of Queen Victoria (London: Muller, 1972):

> "One of the reasons why Victoria continued to bear children was her belief that, by doing so, she kept her grip on Albert . . . . When she was pregnant he was always kind, thoughtful, attentive of her every wish. Here was a problem that he could understand, a train of events to which he could attend. But he knew nothing of the imponderable in women. He was completely inexperienced. He did not appreciate the unreasoned emotions which surged like a maelstrom in Victoria's brain. Albert's answer to all the problems of life was to exercise reason . . . . When Victoria began throwing things and screaming her accusations into his face, he would retire to write a paper on the cause of the outburst. She would then receive a letter beginning, 'Dear Child' and containing simple ingredients for an antidote to emotion. This did not help matters. Albert soon learned that any action that he took at such times was wrong. Answering back led to faster, louder vituperation.

Remaining quiet was classified as insulting. Retiring behind a locked door eventually led to an attack upon its
panels by royal fists.... Even (Lord) Melbourne, a past
master at dealing with women, had on one occasion
quavered and feared to sit down as the fire blazed in the
eyes of the eighteen-year-old queen. A cabinet minister
was known to fly from her presence, too frightened to
follow the rule of withdrawal. Thus Albert looked forward
to the period of pregnancy—it gave emotion a reason."

Prince Albert, Lord Melbourne, and the Cabinet ministers
mentioned above were not as fortunately placed to deal with
premenstrual syndrome as you will be when you have read this
book, especially the new Chapter 11, "Advice to Men."

Premenstrual syndrome knows no geographical, social, racial, or economic boundaries; its sufferings and tragedies are
spread evenly throughout our society. For many it is sufficient
reassurance to know that other normal women also experience
the same monthly feelings, while the knowledge that there is a
satisfactory answer provides them with hope for the future.

1

The Curse of Eve

Once a month women are reminded that their reproductive system is still in the process of evolution. But it is no good waiting another two or three million years for Mother Nature to iron out the flaws. In the short term it is better to try to understand the way our body works, the problems with which the silent majority tries to cope, and how best they can be helped.

The other natural functions of the body, such as growth, respiration, digestion, and excretion, go on day by day without pain. Indeed, if pain is present it is abnormal, a cause for concern, and a thorough search is made to find and eradicate the disease. On the other hand, the two natural feminine physiological processes, menstruation and childbirth, are seldom completely without pain. It is thought that less than one woman in ten goes through her childbearing years without at some time suffering from period pain or premenstrual tension. It is now universally accepted (although it was not always so) that women experiencing pain during labor deserve relief with analgesics and anesthetics. Many even go into training for this one-day event with weekly relaxation classes. One hopes that the days of enlightenment are not too far away when treatment for the relief of period pains and premenstrual problems will be accepted as the natural right of every woman the world over.

Menstruation represents a failed pregnancy, and only occurs if the woman is neither pregnant nor breastfeeding. It was therefore comparatively rare in primitive societies. A normal woman can expect to menstruate once a month for an average of 35 years, but our great-grandmothers, who breastfed their families of 12 children as the only known method of contraception, averaged 11 years of intermittent menstruation. By contrast, today's mother of two, who breastfeeds for an average of 3 months, may expect almost continuous menstrual cycles for 33 years.

> *Anne,* 34 years old, was brought to the doctor's office by her Catholic priest, because of a severe asthma attack that accompanied her last menstruation. She was asked if asthma had also accompanied her previous menstruation before this last one. She took a few minutes to think about it before admitting, "I was only 18 at the time and I can't really remember." She had 14 children, and for the last 16 years had either been pregnant or breastfeeding.

Pain is not the only symptom associated with menstruation: there are also the psychological and bodily symptoms that come out of the blue once a month, usually just before menstruation, and come under the omnibus heading of Premenstrual Syndrome. Examples include Barbara and Carol.

Barbara wrote:

> "I have such drastic changes in personality before a period I think I am going mad. I cannot understand how I can feel so differently toward my children, one day loving and caring for them and the next day being so hateful and rough, being bad-tempered and smacking them for nothing. How guilty I feel when I see my own daughter, aged 5, copying me and smacking her dolls."

Carol wrote:

> "I have one fantastic week each month, but after ovulation my whole body changes, my breasts start to swell, I look five months pregnant with a swollen stomach, my chest

feels tight, and I just can't breathe because of asthma. I usually have a migraine on the first day of menstruation."

Relief is possible for women with painful periods and also for those with premenstrual symptoms, like Barbara and Carol. However, first it is necessary for them to make the connection between their symptoms and menstruation. This means it depends either on the patient herself to recognize it, or else her husband, mother, close friend, or doctor has to. Once the problem is recognized, treatment is available, as we will see in later chapters.

It has been said, "Man is born to suffer, but woman is born to suffer more," and sometimes it seems that no efforts are being made to ease a woman's sufferings. Consider this list of excuses taken from recent letters:

"It's not fatal and doesn't last long"

"She'll get over it"

"Cool it, lady, you're neurotic"

"Things will be easier when you're married" or ". . . when you have had children" or ". . . when the children have grown up"

"Learn to live with it and take more exercise"

"Accept the symptoms—you're not going mad—and learn to relax"

"It's only because you've not enough to do" (*to a woman with three children, all under school age*)

"You're working too hard" (*to a woman with one child at school*)

"You're only trying to jump on the bandwagon like 90% of other women"

And so the excuses go on, with the adoption of an ostrich-like attitude to once-a-month problems, and with no efforts made to solve them.

There is nothing new about these menstrual problems. Hippocrates, the father of medicine, blamed premenstrual tension on "the agitated blood of a woman seeking a way of escape from the womb." Primitive man found it difficult to understand how women could lose blood every month, yet neither be ill nor die. Even today many men are amazed that women can accept the regular loss of blood so cheerfully when they themselves panic each time their nose bleeds or they cut a finger. But women only rarely complain of the bleeding itself; it is how they feel and look, and the pains they suffer, that worry them.

When primitive tribes lived in isolation, there might be only one menstruating woman present at any one time. It was natural then to endow her with supernatural powers normally ascribed to gods. These powers included an ability to stop hailstorms, whirlwinds, and lightning if she went out into the open unclothed. Menstrual blood was also thought to be endowed with valuable properties, such as the power to extinguish fires, temper metals, fashion swords, and protect men against wounds in battle. A thread soaked in menstrual blood was considered a valuable treatment for epilepsy and headache. (Today we often find that once menstruation starts, the premenstrual epilepsy or headache is relieved.)

Myths about menstruation are worldwide. In some parts of the world the presence of a menstruating woman was believed to cause harm, being able to sour wines, blight crops, rust iron or bronze, and turn copper green. She could cause cattle to abort, seeds to dry up, fruit to die on trees, bright mirrors to become dulled, the edge to be taken off sharpened metal, a hive of bees to perish, the strings of harps to break, clocks to stop, and linen to turn black. Can one wonder that women in India went into *purdah* at these times?

During the Middle Ages it was believed that menstruation demonstrated the essential sinfulness and inferiority of women. They were therefore forbidden to attend church or take communion, a custom still observed in the Greek Orthodox Church today. For the same reason, Orthodox Jewish women are instructed to make themselves plain and unattractive during menstruation, to avoid exciting their husbands sexually. Following menstruation, the woman is required to undergo a ritualistic cleansing by immersing herself three times in "a body of water."

In different countries there are local customs associated with menstruation that are concerned chiefly with the local industries and fear of their failure. In Indonesia, menstruating women may not enter tobacco fields or work in rice paddies. In Saigon they may not be employed in opium factories, lest the opium turn bitter. In France and Germany they were excluded from the wineries and breweries lest they turned wine or beer sour; and in the Canary Islands today women are not allowed in the grape-crushing area. In France the presence of a menstruating woman during the boiling process in sugar refineries might turn the sugar black. Parsee women in India may not look at a fire lest their glance extinguish it. In Syria, if pickling is done by menstruating women it is believed the food will be putrefied. In South Africa, menstruating women may not come into contact with cattle for fear the milk will turn sour. Until the last century in England it was believed that if menstruating women salted meat it would not keep.

The problems associated with menstruation are obviously not new; they represent the eternal mystery of women. What is new is the changing attitude of the medical profession, which now contains a few doctors, far too few, who have interested themselves in these problems and have shown that they can be successfully treated, and treated without witchcraft. Other doctors are trying to learn how to correctly diagnose and properly treat these problems, but they are often confused by the bewildering amount of misinformation and, frequently, *wrong* information that is constantly being presented to them by those with little or no practical experience of premenstrual syndrome, or by entrepreneurs looking for financial gain. These doctors see this shamefully neglected subject of menstruation, with its complexity of symptoms that can change a woman from Jekyll to Hyde within minutes, as a challenge to be met.

THE MENSTRUAL CYCLE

To ensure the continuation of the human species, nature has evolved in a woman a system that produces an egg cell at precisely the right time for it to be fertilized by the sperm of the male. Research has shown that this is not the simple process we used to believe; it is really very complex. There is no need for us to go into all the details, however, for nature's basic system is the menstrual cycle which can be explained in quite simple terms and still be a correct account of the process of childbearing.

Woman is born with two ovaries containing thousands of immature egg cells. Each month, in response to a message from the pituitary gland, one of the unripe egg cells develops inside a tiny microscopic ring of cells, which gradually increases to form a little balloon or cyst called the Graafian follicle. These cells make the menstrual hormone, *estrogen*, about which we will be hearing much more later. When the little egg cell is fully developed it appears as a blister on the surface of the ovary, and under a further message from the pituitary gland it bursts and releases the mature egg cell. This is known as *ovulation*. The egg cell makes its way down the fallopian tubes to the womb, a journey that takes about 14 days. Meanwhile, the yellow scar tissue left behind when the blister bursts fills up with new cells that produce the second important menstrual hormone, *progesterone*. The progesterone acts on the lining of the womb to turn it into a soft, spongy layer in which the fertilized egg cell can embed itself if a pregnancy occurs.

During intercourse millions of male sperm are projected into the vagina and journey through the womb up into one of the fallopian tubes in an attempt to fertilize the egg cell, so that conception will occur and pregnancy can begin. The fertilized egg passes into the womb and becomes embedded in the new soft lining, where it develops into a baby. Following successful fertilization, progesterone will continue to be produced to protect the developing baby from being rejected by the mother's womb. However, if the egg cell has not been fertilized, the production of progesterone begins to fall. About 14 days after ovulation the soft, spongy lining of the womb, which is then not needed, disintegrates and is shed, together with the unfertilized egg cell. This is menstruation, which represents a failed pregnancy.

WE ARE ALL DIFFERENT

Women are different in so many ways: personal and facial characteristics, personality, parentage, family size and position, environment, education, previous illnesses, reactions to food and to drugs. So it is no surprise to realize that women are also different in their menstrual pattern and their reaction to menstrual symptoms.

Men are also different. The range of responses shown by men to women with premenstrual syndrome and menstrual problems runs the gamut from genuine sympathy and understanding to annoyance, amazement, anger, aggression, disbelief, ridicule, and withdrawal. There is even the partner who says, "You've had it long enough, you ought to know how to deal with it." (See Chapter 11.)

NORMAL VARIATIONS OF MENSTRUATION

Each woman's menstrual cycle is unique and individual, so there are considerable variations. The menstrual flow, which is the disintegrated lining of the womb, may appear as a pink watery discharge, or as thick red blood. It may be reddish-brown or black, and it may contain shreds or small blood clots. All these variations are normal and healthy. Similarly, menstruation may occur every 21 or every 36 days, or anywhere in between, and it will still be considered normal and compatible with full reproductive functioning. A variation of 4 days in the length of a woman's cycle month to month is also normal and almost to be expected. Ovulation occurs no earlier than 14 days before menstruation so, taking into account the different lengths of menstrual cycles, ovulation can occur as early as day 10 in a 21-day cycle or as late as day 22 in a 36-day cycle.

This variation in the length of the menstrual cycle is also important in determining the timing of medication for menstrual problems. Some treatments for premenstrual syndrome suggest starting on day 12 and continuing until day 26, but this is of little value to the woman with a 36-day cycle, who then receives no medication during the vital last 10 days of her cycle. From all this it is obvious that there can be no standard dose or timing of treatment that will be appropriate to every woman suffering from premenstrual syndrome. Each woman requires a personal regimen of treatment for success.

There are also variations in the amount of menstrual flow on different days of menstruation. Some women have the heaviest flow on the first, second, and third day and then stop abruptly. Others have moderate loss for a day or two and then the heaviest loss on the third or fourth day. Then there are those women who have a scanty loss for a day or two, with the flow gradually increasing in amount. It is important for the doctor to know the day of heaviest loss, because in premenstrual syndrome the spontaneous relief of symptoms will not occur until the day of heaviest loss. This means that for some women symptoms may well occur during the early days of menstruation.

PHASES OF THE MENSTRUAL CYCLE

The menstrual cycles of different women vary considerably in length, but for the purpose of understanding the hormonal changes during the menstrual cycle, it is convenient to divide it into seven phases of 4 days each, which assumes the woman has a precise cycle of 28 days. In the seven phases there are no two phases that have the same levels of hormones circulating in the blood. (See Figure 1.)

The phases are:

Days 1– 4   *Menstruation*, with rising estrogen levels

Days 5– 8   *Postmenstruum*, with peak estrogen levels

Days 9–12   *Late postmenstruum*, with falling estrogen levels

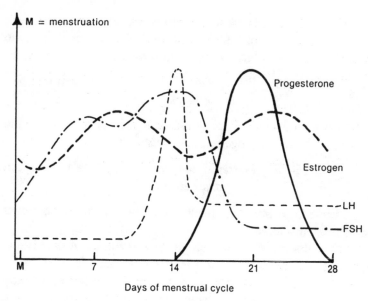

Figure 1 Menstrual hormone variations during the menstrual cycle

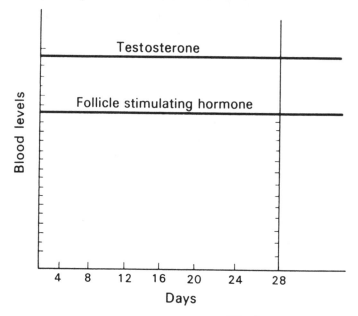

Figure 2 Male hormone levels during a month

Days 13–16   *Ovulation*, with low estrogen and peak levels of follicle stimulating hormones (FSH) and luteinising hormones (LH)

Days 17–20   *Post-ovulation*, with rising estrogen and progesterone levels

Days 21–24   *Early premenstruum*, with peak estrogen and progesterone levels

Days 25–28   *Premenstruum*, with falling levels of estrogen and progesterone.

For comparison the steady daily levels of male hormones are shown in Figure 2.

The first 4 days of menstruation and the last 4 days before menstruation are known as the *paramenstruum*. It is a useful term that is often used in surveys, for these days occur regardless of the length of a woman's cycle. Any adjustment needed due to a cycle being longer or shorter than 28 days is made in the late postmenstruum. In long cycles the postmenstruum will be longer than 8 days, while short cycles will have a short postmenstruum.

Readers should note that the progesterone that is present from ovulation until menstruation is a natural hormone, not to be confused with the man-made progestogens or progestins found in the pill, which have completely different actions. (See also pages 208–210.)

The attitudes of women to regular menstruation vary considerably. Some think of it as a sign of normalcy and an indication of good health. Others regard it as a sign of femininity with maternal attributes, or an assurance that though they are not pregnant now, they are fertile. Menopausal women see menstruation as a sign of their youthfulness to which they are so anxious to cling, while those who see menstruation as a once-a-month nuisance, to be tolerated as Mother Nature's wish, wonder why medical scientists have not given more thought to the abolition of the associated ailments and complaints.

A study of the words used throughout the world to describe menstruation is fascinating. In Jamaica, Nigeria, Egypt, and Mexico, words are used that imply a state of ill-health or pain, such as "being unwell" or "having the blues." In Yugoslavia, Mexico, Egypt, and the Philippines, the menstrual bleeding is often personified as a "visitor," while in Britain it may be called "the curse," or given the familiarity of an old friend like "Charlie," or "Archie." In Nigeria and Jamaica, young girls are taught about growing up using the analogy of "flowers and bees," so that when menstruation occurs it is called "flowers." Women in Egypt and Korea often use terms associated with sanitary pads and bathing. In Indonesia the words used are associated with pollution or with purification. In the Philippines, the phrase "desire for abortion" is sometimes used when describing menstruation.

Psychologists object to the use of the word "curse," claiming that it conditions women to expect trouble with menstruation. On the other hand, women have as many menstrual problems in Nigeria and Jamaica, where the word "flowers" is used. There is no doubt that psychological factors do play a part in menstrual problems, but this is only secondary to the hormonal effects.

2

Mood Swings

"Tell me, Doctor, why does my wife, who is usually very warm and loving, become angry and totally impossible for no obvious reason once a month?"

There are innumerable answers to that question. Usually, the blame is laid on external events, while the chemical upheaval that occurs within her body at the time of menstruation is overlooked. These chemical changes can produce changes in personality or sudden mood swings as menstruation approaches, followed by a return to normalcy as soon as or shortly after the menstrual flow starts. This is known as premenstrual syndrome or, more familiarly, as PMS. (Doctors use the word "syndrome" for a group of complaints or symptoms that cluster together.)

The mood swings may vary from being a minor nuisance to causing a major disturbance. There may just be an unexpected reaction to a trivial irritation, a hilarious conversation abruptly ended by a cutting remark or a blunt rebuke, or a loss of a sense of humor. On the other end of the scale there may be violent verbal and physical abuse, or smashing and throwing of things. At the far extreme lies the possibility of suicide, homicide, or infanticide. It is easy for an observer to attribute this to a lack of self-control, or call it a temperamental outburst, or blame the woman's character. Too rarely are these mood swings properly attributed to the natural ebb and flow of the menstrual hormones, over which the woman has so little control.

These premenstrual mood swings are widespread and occur in at least half of all women. This means that there is also another 50% of women who do not experience them at all, and do not know what the other half are suffering. Why this fortunate 50% do not suffer is explained in Chapter 17. Men, too, do not experience such changes in hormone levels. The male sex hormones remain on an even keel day by day throughout the month, as shown by the levels of follicle stimulating hormone and testosterone in Figure 2. How different are the levels of the woman's four sex hormones, *follicle stimulating hormone, luteinising hormone, estrogen, and progesterone*, which vary daily throughout the month, as shown in Figure 1. Only a slight imbalance in any of these levels is enough to cause problems for a woman.

The term "Premenstrual Syndrome" is used to embrace *any symptoms or complaints that regularly come just before or during early menstruation, but are absent at other times of the cycle*. It is a precise definition, and means that the symptoms must be present each and every month. Symptoms must occur premenstrually, and there must be a symptom-free phase each cycle. It is the absence of symptoms after menstruation that is so important in this definition.

There is an endless list of some 150 different symptoms that may occur in this syndrome, including tension, depression, tiredness, irritability, backache, asthma, sinusitis, epilepsy, and weight-gain. Fortunately, no woman suffers from all the possible symptoms. All of these symptoms can also be experienced by men, but in the male they are random complaints that do not occur once every month. It is only in women that we find these symptoms occurring cyclically and regularly related to menstruation.

Premenstrual syndrome needs to be differentiated from *menstrual distress*. Menstrual distress covers *symptoms present throughout the menstrual cycle, with increased intensity before or during menstruation*. Such symptoms may be intermittent, as with headaches, or continuously present throughout the day, as with anxiety or depression. It is unfortunately true that in all chronic diseases (for instance, rheumatoid arthritis, bronchitis, multiple sclerosis, schizophrenia, glaucoma) women find their symptoms increase before menstruation.

Most women with premenstrual syndrome suffer from more than one symptom at the same time. For instance, many sufferers will notice weight-gain and an increase in tension before the onset of a premenstrual headache. Removing one symptom, for example by giving a tranquilizer to ease the tension, is of little help to the gain in weight and the headache.

It is also important to remember that the definition of premenstrual syndrome requires not only the presence of symptoms related to menstruation, but also the complete absence of these symptoms at other times of the menstrual cycle. It is the absence of symptoms and the change of mood after menstruation back to a happier, energetic feeling of normalcy that clinches the diagnosis.

This letter from a patient illustrates the point:

"I suffered from the usual premenstrual symptoms for five years, and my tension, irritability, and depression were blamed on nerves. I must say I could never understand this, as it was only at certain times of the month that I seemed to be so nervous, tense, depressed, and lacking in confidence. I found that about 10 to 12 days before my period I felt as if something was draining out of me, and as if something chemical was happening. So often I tried to pull myself together at this time and it just never worked. I get so irritable and nervous a week before menstruation that I just want to shut myself up in the house; I feel as if I can't go out to work, and I avoid any sort of social engagement at this time of the month. At other times I'm O.K."

The exact type and severity of symptoms vary with each individual, but every sufferer's schedule of discomfort is the same, month by month, or rather, cycle by cycle. The easiest tool for recognizing the relationship of symptoms to menstruation and the absence of symptoms at other times of the cycle is the simple menstrual chart shown in Figure 3 and discussed in Chapter 3.

The start of the mood swings may be quite sudden, and the victim may surprise even herself by her outrageous behavior. One person described it as "a blanket of fog that enfolds me," while a 20-year-old student thought of it as "changing from high gear to low in the car." In other cases the beginning may be quite gradual, with symptoms becoming worse day by day. Problems may start at ovulation and last the full 14 days until menstruation, so that one sufferer felt she had been "crazy for half my life," or they may occur only days or hours before the onset of menstruation. Even if they only last for a few days, they can be a source of great anguish, as one letter-writer described:

> "Every month it is the same, and the thought of being knocked out for a couple of days each month for the next 20 or so years fills me with desperation. It is such a complete waste of days that could be used for living instead of for feeling trapped."

In premenstrual epilepsy the attack may be measured in minutes or hours rather than in days, though the symptoms tend to last longer as one approaches menopause. A 42-year-old teacher wondered if "this gradual lengthening of the negative mood means that pretty soon there may be no bright spell left at all." It was good to be able to reassure her that, however long the premenstrual mood lasts, there is always a bright spell once a month after menstruation, because premenstrual symptoms do not start earlier than 14 days before menstruation, regardless of how long or short the menstrual cycle may be.

For many women the onset of menstruation works like a charm, and the relief that comes as the blood flows has been likened to "a cloud lifting," or the "curtain opening again." An occasional sufferer may even be freed from her symptoms a day or a few hours before menstruation starts. Yet others find relief is slower and comes only with the full menstrual flow. If there is only slight spotting of blood for one, two, or more days at the beginning, they will not get relief of symptoms until this changes to a full menstrual flow. Indeed, their worst time may be during those early days of spotting, and they may not regain their joy of living until a couple of days after menstruation has finished.

When it's over, one may hear a loving husband announce, "She's now like the woman I married!"

Age and pregnancy are two factors that tend to make the symptoms of premenstrual syndrome become worse and last longer, so it may be first diagnosed when a woman is in her thirties. In fact, in 1963 Dr. T. Stacy Lloyd of Virginia suggested the name "Mid-Thirties Syndrome" for this same collection of symptoms. By their mid-thirties many women have been married, been on the pill and stopped, and many have had their pregnancies and possibly been sterilized. All of these are factors that increase the incidence and severity of premenstrual syndrome. At the International Symposium on Premenstrual Syndrome held in South Carolina in 1983 many speakers, when presenting their papers, mentioned the age of the patients they had studied, and these were invariably in their mid-thirties. These were women who had visited premenstrual syndrome clinics and had been diagnosed as suffering from the disease. But all too often it is the young adolescents and those in their early twenties who suffer in silence without being diagnosed. Instead they are thought to be ill-tempered, miserable, and lazy; they are unloved, and so end up alienated, leading to yet more problems. Fortunately, the term "Mid-Thirties Syndrome" never caught on, and hopefully it will be forgotten, as it is unfair to those in other age groups.

The increase in severity of symptoms is more marked in the years just before menopause, so much so that premenstrual mood swings are often blamed on menopause. A 50-year-old woman exclaimed, "I've been in menopause for the last 15 years—when will it ever end?" It is more than likely that she had been suffering from undiagnosed premenstrual syndrome for all that time.

Fortunately, there is an end to this exclusively feminine syndrome. When the menopausal changes are complete, menstruation ends and so do the monthly fluctuations of mood and other symptoms. Menopause marks the end of childbearing. Ovulation ceases, and gradually women's hormones readjust. This is the time when one may look forward to an era of serenity.

3

————————— ✿ —————————

Clearing the Confusion

Without a doubt, there is much confusion about premenstrual syndrome. Medical professionals are confounded by it, whether they are gynecologists, psychiatrists, or endocrinologists. Even general practitioners, who see the condition first and are in an ideal situation for treating it, are equally perplexed. Few specialists know anything about it, even though premenstrual syndrome invades every specialty. Add to this the abysmal lack of knowledge and experience of premenstrual syndrome revealed in the writings of an increasing number of lay authors, together with the appalling ignorance and utter befuddlement of the media's presentation on the subject and it is only too easy to understand how the bewilderment continues to grow. Hopefully, this chapter will clear away these mists of confusion.

First, it is essential to establish a definition of the disease in question in order to achieve a proper diagnosis. The definition of premenstrual syndrome is "the presence of any symptoms or complaints that regularly come just before or during early menstruation, but are absent at other times of the cycle." This precise definition means that three requirements must be fulfilled for a correct diagnosis:

1) Symptoms must be present every month for at least the previous 3 months

2) Symptoms must be present premenstrually, and cannot start before ovulation

3) There must be complete absence of symptoms after menstruation for a minimum of 7 days.

The successful treatment of any disease depends on the accuracy of the diagnosis. To achieve that accuracy, a doctor must take three things into consideration: symptoms, signs, and investigations. That means the doctor listens to the patient's account of the complaint, takes note of any signs of disease that may be revealed by examination, and studies the results of blood tests, X rays, and other investigations. The doctor accepts the patient's account of her symptoms (be they a sore throat or a pain in some part of the body), and after examining for signs and considering the results of tests, makes the diagnosis and treats her accordingly. All too often, when women come to their doctor claiming they have premenstrual symptoms, the doctor accepts their claim at face value without appreciating the need to check the diagnosis further before giving treatment.

TIME RELATIONSHIP OF SYMPTOMS TO MENSTRUATION

The doctor must verify the diagnosis of premenstrual syndrome, because there are no special symptoms indicative of the disease. The disease only affects women of childbearing age, but all the symptoms can be complained of by men, children, and post-menopausal women. There are no specific signs discovered on examination and no definitive investigations. How, then, to make an accurate diagnosis of a disease that has no special symptoms, no specific signs, and no distinctive investigations? The one clear diagnostic clue is the time relationship of symptoms to menstruation. It is therefore necessary to find a new method of diagnosis that enables this critical time relationship to be clearly established.

Psychiatrists frequently use questionnaires as part of their diagnostic procedures, asking the patient numerous questions and analyzing the replies. This is a useful method. It allows numerical scores to be obtained for an individual's level of depression, anxiety, neuroticism, or marital stability. This score can then be used to compare the results of different treatments.

MENSTRUAL DISTRESS QUESTIONNAIRES

In 1968 Rudolph Moos designed a questionnaire which is very effective in demonstrating the amount of distress caused by menstruation, although it cannot differentiate premenstrual syndrome from menstrual pain or distress. In the Moos Menstrual Distress Questionnaire a woman is asked to complete 47 different questions each night on a six-point scale. These include questions such as "Today did you have any orderliness? . . . excitement? . . . loneliness?" It is a method that relies on the honesty, reliability, and determination of the candidate. While it may be easy to carefully consider your reply and complete the questionnaire for one—or even seven—consecutive days, one doubts the accuracy of the responses when, as in the tests conducted by Dr. Sampson in 1978 and 1988, women were asked to complete a questionnaire every single day for 6 months. Moreover, there is always a need for caution in interpreting the results of questionnaires when they are used for purposes other than those for which they were designed.

Unfortunately, the Moos Questionnaires concentrate on common psychiatric symptoms and do not cover all the possible 150 symptoms that may occur in premenstrual syndrome. Some useful questions that are missing include, "Did you shoplift today?" "Did you have too much alcohol today?" "How many puffs of your inhaler did you need to control your asthma?" "Could you wear your contact lenses today?" Furthermore, the questionnaires cannot be answered by those few severely ill patients who are temporarily confused, deluded, or hallucinating during the premenstruum, but are free of symptoms during the postmenstruum.

It must not be forgotten that the information obtained on such questionnaires needs to be prospective, obtained daily, rather than retrospective, obtained by such questions as, "During the days before menstruation do you suffer from . . . ?" Today, women have been educated by the media to know that head-aches, bloatedness, backache, and irritability tend to occur pre-menstrually. If they suffer from these symptoms at all, they may automatically assume that their headaches or other symptoms occurred premenstrually.

THE MENSTRUAL CHART

If the help of the patient is needed in making the diagnosis, it is important to keep the diagnostic aids simple to eliminate the possibility of inaccuracy and guesswork. The menstrual chart shown in Figure 3 is widely used by doctors, and is easy enough for anyone to copy. The purpose of the chart is to provide the precise information necessary to make an accurate diagnosis of premenstrual syndrome. This is done by recording the actual dates of menstruation and the days when symptoms or com-plaints are present. The woman is asked to choose only her most important symptoms—those complaints she would most like to lose. These symptoms are then given symbols, such as "H" for headache, "X" for quarrels, "T" for tension. A small "h," "x," or "t" can be used for mild symptoms, and capital letters for symp-toms that are really severe. There shouldn't be a need to use more than one letter for any one symptom. It doesn't matter what letters are used; for example, the letter "M" may be used to represent menstruation, but some use "P" for period. The chart is completed each night with a record of whether the symptom was present or absent, and whether it was severe dur-ing that day. Some women like to insert a dot on those days when they feel well; this ensures that they complete the record. The chart should be completed daily regardless of the phase of the menstrual cycle or the apparent cause of the symptom. Doc-tors interpreting the chart are quite aware that external cir-cumstances may cause the same symptoms. For instance, a few hours spent watching your child having his lacerated leg sutured in an emergency room will cause you to feel tense, irritable, or depressed, regardless of the phase of the cycle. And, you may have every reason to feel exhausted or have a headache after an all-night delayed flight returning from a vacation.

Name _____ Year _____

	Jan.	Feb.	Mar.	Apr.	May	Jun.	Jul.	Aug.	Sep.	Oct.	Nov.	Dec.
1												
2												
3												
4												
5												
6												
7												
8												
9												
10												
11												
12												
13												
14												
15												
16												
17												
18												
19												
20												
21												
22												
23												
24												
25												
26												
27												
28												
29												
30												
31												

Figure 3   A simple menstrual chart

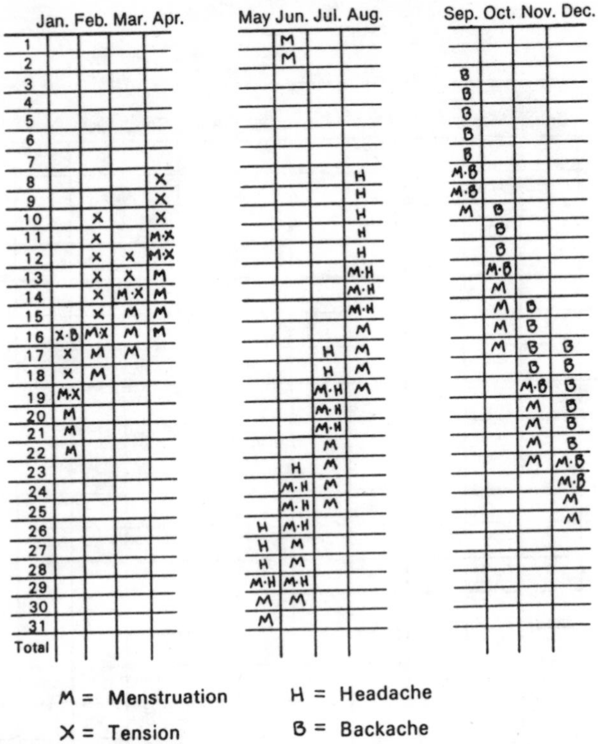

	Jan.	Feb.	Mar.	Apr.	May	Jun.	Jul.	Aug.	Sep.	Oct.	Nov.	Dec.
1					M							
2					M							
3									B			
4									B			
5									B			
6									B			
7									B			
8				X			H		M·B			
9				X			H		M·B			
10		X		X			H		M	B		
11		x		M·X			H			B		
12		x	x	M·X			H			B		
13		x	X	M			M·H			M·B		
14		x	M·X	M			M·H			M		
15		x	M	M			M·H			M	B	
16	X·B	MX	M	M			M			M	B	
17	x	M	M			H	M			M	B	B
18	x	M				H	M				B	B
19	M·X					M·H	M				M·B	B
20	M					M·H	M				M	B
21	M						M·H				M	B
22	M						M				M	B
23						H	M				M	M·B
24						M·H	M					M·B
25						M·H	M					M
26					H	M·H						
27					H	M						
28					H	M						
29					M·H	M·H						
30					M	M						
31					M							
Total												

M = Menstruation   H = Headache

X = Tension   B = Backache

Figure 4   Menstrual charts diagnostic of premenstrual syndrome

From a menstrual chart it immediately becomes obvious whether symptoms are clustered around menstruation, as in Figure 4, or occur haphazardly throughout the month, as in Figure 5. It is easy to see the duration of menstruation or of symptoms, and whether the menstrual cycle is short, for the "M"s will be going up the chart, or long, for the "M"s will be going down the chart. It is also not necessary for the woman to be menstruating to obtain information about the cyclical character of her symptoms. Cyclical symptoms can occur even before menstruation has begun, at times of occasional missed menstruation, at menopause, or after removal of the womb or ovaries.

One mother, a sales executive who was herself receiving treatment for premenstrual syndrome, was disturbed to find that

	Jan.	Feb.	Mar.	Apr.	May	Jun.	Jul.	Aug.
1	X		X	M				H
2			X	M				
3			X	M	H	H		
4								
5				X				H
6				X	H	H		
7			M		H			
8	X		M·X			H		
9	X		M			H		
10		X	M			H		
11								H
12		M			M	H		
13		M	X	X	M			
14		M			M·H	H		
15		X			M	M		
16	X				M	M		
17	M				M		M	
18	M				M	M	M	M
19	M	X			M	M	M	M
20		X		X		M	M	M
21			X			M	M	M
22			X		H	M		M
23	X				H	M		
24	X					M·H		
25	X							
26		X						
27				X				
28			X	M	H			H
29				M		H		
30	X			M			H	
31					H			
Total								

M = Menstruation   X = Quarrels

H = Headaches

Figure 5   Menstrual chart with unrelated symptoms

her 13-year-old daughter had occasional "off" days when she was rude and lazy, which was quite out of character for her. Then the mother received reports from school indicating that the girl had occasional rebellious days during which she found it hard to accept discipline. The mother carefully recorded the dates of these problems (shown on the chart in Figure 6), which occurred at intervals of 32–36 days. When the daughter later started to menstruate, the timing of her menstrual cycle averaged 35 days. What had happened was that this mother had diagnosed her daughter's premenstrual syndrome before menstru-

	Jan.	Feb.	Mar.	Apr.	May	Jun.
1					X	
2						X
3						X
4						
5						X
6						
7						
8						
9						
10						
11						
12						
13						
14						
15						
16	X					
17	X	X				
18	X	X				
19						
20		X				
21	X	X				
22						
23		X				
24			X			
25			X			
26				X		
27			X	X		
28				X		
29			X	X		
30			X			
31					X	
Total						

Figure 6   Chart of adolescent girl with cyclical symptoms before the start of menstruation

ation had started. It is not necessary for menstruation or ovulation to occur before PMS develops.

If the chart does not show a relationship of symptoms to menstruation, there is no point in trying to make it fit the PMS pattern. It is wiser to show the chart to your doctor, as it may contain valuable clues that will indicate the true problem. It is not unknown for some women to copy a chart straight from a book and then ask for help; unfortunately, in these circumstances there is little the doctor can do to help.

Occasionally, the diagnosis may be made by others, whose observations reveal the cyclical character of the symptoms. For instance, a legal executive noted the days when her secretary's typing deteriorated and she became aggressive. When these revealed a pattern of recurring every 30–33 days, the boss advised her secretary to get medical help. The value of similar information received from police, prison officers, and medical records is discussed in Chapter 15.

HORMONE BLOOD TESTS

Tests to determine the blood level of progesterone are of little value in the diagnosis of premenstrual syndrome. The secretion of progesterone from the corpus luteum of the ovary is intermittent and changes with marked variations within 30 minutes, so single blood samples taken on one day are of no help. Also, low levels of progesterone are found in women who are not ovulating, although they do not necessarily suffer from premenstrual syndrome. However, a blood test to estimate the binding capacity of sex hormone binding globulin (SHBG) has proved valuable in diagnosing premenstrual syndrome. My daughter, Dr. Maureen Dalton, showed in 1981 that 50 women suffering from severe, well-diagnosed premenstrual syndrome all had SHBG-binding levels below normal, compared with 50 healthy women who were adamant they did not suffer any premenstrual symptoms. (See Figure 7.) Furthermore, her tests showed that SHBG levels rise when progesterone is administered, and the greater the dose of progesterone the higher the SHBG level. (See Figure 8.) Later work showed that if progestogens were administered, the SHBG levels were lowered.

There are limitations on this test's usefulness, however, for the woman whose blood is to be tested must be free from all medication (which includes analgesics, oral contraceptives, laxatives, and vitamin preparations), must not be unduly obese or excessively hairy, and should not suffer from liver or thyroid disease. Furthermore, the blood must be centrifuged and stored frozen until analyzed by an elaborate method, which is available only at a few specialized testing centers.

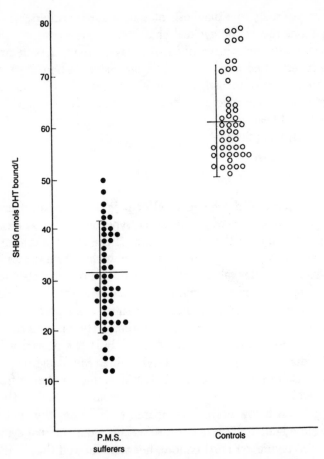

Figure 7   SHBG-binding capacity in 50 patients with severe
premenstrual syndrome compared with 50
symptom-free controls

DIAGNOSTIC POINTERS

Before a diagnosis of premenstrual syndrome can be made,
women must complete the menstrual chart for 2 or 3 months.
When selecting women for clinical trials on PMS, the 2-month
daily recording is the minimum, but sometimes a rough diagnosis is needed earlier. This can be done by considering characteristics that are common to most women with premenstrual

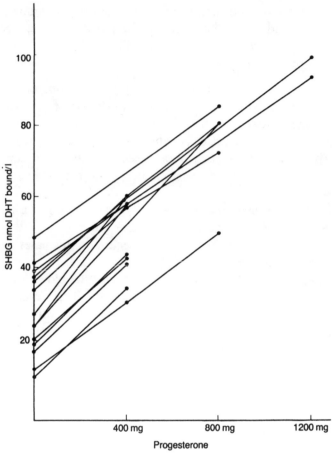

Figure 8   Effect of progesterone on SHBG levels

syndrome, and that differentiate them from those who do not suffer from PMS. These characteristics are usually referred to as "diagnostic pointers." The rest of this chapter will deal with these characteristics and their usefulness as diagnostic pointers.

Medical students are taught that the onset of premenstrual syndrome is linked with P-P-P-A: **puberty, pregnancy, the pill,** and **amenorrhea,** or absence of menstruation, such as occurs after anorexia nervosa or after serious illnesses or accidents. In the young adolescent, premenstrual syndrome may result in an unexpected change of personality. One mother wrote:

"For three weeks of the month our daughter is charming, capable, and intelligent, then for the few days before her period she is sharp-tongued, impossible to live with, and seems to be boiling with rage."

Spasmodic dysmenorrhea, or severe period pain, occurs only in ovulatory cycles and is unusual in sufferers of premenstrual syndrome. (See Chapter 8.) On the other hand, because their early **periods** are practically painless and uneventful, many young women with premenstrual syndrome initially fail to connect the symptoms in other parts of their body with menstruation.

Menstruation may stop unexpectedly when dieting, during a serious illness or accident, or when under great stress. When menstruation restarts, PMS frequently begins, or increases in severity. (See *Amenorrhea*, pages 158–160.)

During pregnancy menstruation stops, and the blood level of progesterone rises to 30–50 times the peak level reached during the premenstruum. At this time most women with premenstrual syndrome lose their symptoms. But even in symptom-free women, premenstrual syndrome may develop unexpectedly when menstruation returns after a pregnancy. If the pregnancy has been complicated by high blood pressure, swelling of the ankles, or an abnormally large gain in weight (signs of preeclamptic toxemia), or if it has been followed by postpartum or postnatal depression, then the chances are high, 10 to 1, that unpleasant premenstrual symptoms will follow in its wake. What is worse, the symptoms are likely to increase in severity after each pregnancy, even if the later pregnancies are normal.

Premenstrual syndrome may start when the woman is on **the pill,** or during the week when she is off it, but complaints are likely to be more marked and the bright and dull days more accentuated when pill-taking ends and the woman resumes her normal menstrual cycle. This cycle may well be 3 or 5 weeks, and not the precise 28 days ordained by the makers of the pill.

Marriage or the beginning of a relationship is often mentioned as another time when PMS starts, but it may be that the partner notices mood swings and other symptoms and relates them to menstruation, while the woman had not noticed the connection earlier. Again, pill-taking may have coincided with marriage.

It is often an outside observer who first notices the mood swings, usually the husband or mother, but occasionally an employer, social worker, friend, or daughter. Following a television broadcast on premenstrual syndrome, a husband wrote:

> "I was so startled to recognize in all these cases the symptoms from which my wife has been suffering for the past eight years. The connection with the menstrual cycle may seem less direct but nevertheless her symptoms are heightened in the premenstrual period and free thereafter. Briefly, they include acute anxiety and depression (in any order, as it seems impossible to distinguish cause and effect) manifested by physical symptoms of pressure on the head (variously described as an iron band around the head or a heavy weight at the back of the head) and dizziness; and by psychological symptoms such as agoraphobia, panic, guilt, obsessions, and depression, sometimes to the extent of feeling suicidal."

Recently it has been recognized that premenstrual syndrome often increases in intensity following tubal ligation. Radwanska, Hammond, and Berger of the University of Illinois showed that after women had the simple operation to block their fallopian tubes, they subsequently produced less progesterone from their ovaries.

During adult life PMS sufferers tend to have large weight swings exceeding 28 pounds, although swings of 50 or more pounds are not unusual. The lowest weight since leaving school is subtracted from the highest non-pregnant weight to measure the adult weight swing. It is irrelevant whether the individual is obese or slim at the time she is weighed.

PMS sufferers have difficulty in going long intervals without food, especially in the premenstruum. When they do, they may get faint, excessively tired, panicky, or irritable. They also tend to suffer from uncontrollable premenstrual food cravings and binges, especially when they have deliberately not eaten for a long time or when they have been dieting. This is not a personality failure but is the result of the hormonal factor. It even occurs in baboons in the jungle, who go up into trees and in isolation gorge on unlimited amounts of honey during their premenstruum.

Tolerance to alcohol also varies during the cycle in premenstrual syndrome sufferers. Although they can usually enjoy their favorite drink with no ill effects, during the premenstruum even a reduced amount causes intoxication.

ᵺ

If a woman gives many positive answers to the diagnostic pointers listed above, there is every likelihood that in 2 months she will return with a positive chart. There are occasions when it may be worth giving a patient a therapeutic trial with progesterone without waiting for a definitive diagnosis, but both the doctor and the patient should be aware that a positive diagnosis has not been made and the patient should not be included in a clinical trial.

An analysis was made of the final diagnosis in over 200 women who attended a premenstrual clinic. Its conclusions were that while the menstrual chart is the only reliable diagnostic method for premenstrual syndrome, the SHBG estimation was more specific, more sensitive, and had a greater predictive value than the checklist score of diagnostic pointers.

4

Premenstrual Tension

Tension may be described in many ways, but the tension that occurs in premenstrual syndrome has three parts to it: depression, tiredness, and irritability. These three aspects are always present in premenstrual tension, although one of them may be more obvious than the others, if only temporarily. Dr. Billig, in 1952, described the depression as "the world looks like a sour apple," the tiredness as "a fall in energy," and the irritability as "feeling crabby"—and there are plenty of women who know exactly what he meant.

These three symptoms may be interwoven, with each one creating equal stress, as *Dorothy's* letter shows:

"Premenstrual tension has been present throughout my reproductive life. I have seen my doctor many times but he has really been unable to help. Perhaps predictably, the condition had grown steadily worse in the years just before my marriage break-up, and has been much, much worse since. The strain is very great and practically unbearable during the premenstrual time. I do not abuse my children physically, but I do verbally, and I think that that can be almost as damaging, although I do try to explain to them why I behave the way I do, and apologize for it. The trouble begins as early as 12 to 14 days after the beginning of the last period, and the first sign is a disturbance of sleep. I get violent dreams and often wake up at night. When it is time to get up, I feel as though I have had no rest at all. Then I become so tense I positively shake, and am so nervous and irritable that I am sorry for anyone who has to live with me. Quite often my heart starts to pound for no obvious reason, though I have not been running or doing heavy exercise. I feel listless and apathetic and often fall asleep during the day. On the other hand, the other half of the cycle I sleep perfectly soundly, and I am energetic, hard-working, and clearheaded. The onset of my period releases the tension, but triggers off headaches that fluctuate from day to day for a couple of days. I cry at the drop of a hat during all this time, and find it hard to deal with any problems objectively. Although I have been very depressed sometimes, I have never had a breakdown, thanks probably to good professional help. Apart from this misery, the rest of the month I am healthy, active, and very rarely ill."

Premenstrual tension, usually abbreviated as "PMT," is only one aspect of premenstrual syndrome, which includes the bodily, physical, or somatic symptoms as well as the psychological ones. Some try to cope with it alone. A competent boutique manager wrote:

"For many years I have managed to keep my PMT a secret, but increasingly I have found it more difficult to suppress. Friends have commented on unexpected changes in my behavior and totally irrational responses to situations. I feel desperate and helpless that I am no longer able to manage my PMT, but it has become a dominant factor in my life today. Normally, I am quite a positive and optimistic person."

The tension may come on quite suddenly, with an inability to relax and feeling generally uptight. One woman complained that when she was in this state she trembled so much that she had difficulty even threading a needle. Frequently, women are shy about mentioning premenstrual tension to their doctor, thinking that it is a common and minor complaint. Instead they use what is known by the medical profession as a "passport symptom"—a somatic symptom like a headache, backache, or flu, which they consider is more acceptable. One mother wrote:

> "When I go to the doctor I am always conscious that I am not physically ill, and so I do not want to tell him all my seemingly petty feelings. After all, one does not want to admit being a failure as a wife and mother."

Sometimes the tension reaches almost manic proportions, with such agitation and restless energy that the woman cannot calm down; she keeps walking up and down, or won't stop talking and just repeats herself endlessly. One husband was upset because:

> "It's no use trying to tell her to relax, she just keeps repeating herself and won't stop talking. New thoughts keep tumbling out. She accuses me of all sorts of things. She just goes on and on and on."

Premenstrual tension, like all other symptoms of premenstrual syndrome, is always aggravated by other stress. None of us can be totally free from stress in our daily life. Work may be more demanding some days because co-workers are absent, or a friend or neighbor may be involved in an accident. The usual effect of these stresses will be an increase in premenstrual tension when the next menstruation approaches. On the other hand, good news will tend to ease the tension, and of course a winning lottery ticket can be most beneficial in relieving premenstrual tension—though only for a month or two!

DEPRESSION

This may be so mild that the word "depression" is not used, or is even denied. For example, the woman may say that she is "fed up" or "feeling down," that she can't laugh easily and has difficulty smiling, or that the whole world is against her and nobody cares. Or the depression may range to the other extreme, with a black cloud hanging over everything, interfering with concentration, so that even simple tasks like reading or playing board games become impossible, and there is the ever-present possibility of suicide.

This risk of possible suicide should always be fully appreciated. One husband wrote describing his wife's depression:

"I feel her life is at risk; she dreads these times so much it colors her whole life. She feels there is no hope."

And a mother described her 20-year-old daughter's depression:

"These occurrences are so regular that for years I have associated them with periods. But when she goes to her doctor, usually in a state of panic, she is either told to pull herself together or given tranquilizers. On at least three occasions she has taken the whole bottle and has had to have her stomach pumped. When she is in this state, she often becomes violent and smashes things or fights with her boyfriend. She may consume vast quantities of alcohol and then try to cut her wrists, always in the wrong direction. After the period, when she is herself, she is such a nice, kind, and good-natured person."

A Washington, D.C., secretary ended her full description of premenstrual depression with the statement:

"The sad thing is that although suicidal thoughts cross my mind at this time, I am a very happy person ordinarily."

The MacKinnons, a husband-and-wife team of doctors, showed as long ago as 1956 that successful suicides predominated during the premenstruum. Studies of attempted suicides in hospitals in London and Delhi, and among the Samaritans in Los Angeles, have all confirmed that half of all women's attempts at suicide are made during the 4 days immediately before or the first 4 days of menstruation.

Although women make more suicide attempts than men, men succeed more frequently. This difference gradually disappears after the age of 50. Dr. John Pollitt, speaking at the Royal Society of Medicine in 1976, suggested that:

"... perhaps one reason for the female's lack of success is that the majority of attempts are made during the premenstrual phase or menstruation. Killing oneself is not easy; success requires careful planning. Women in the premenstrual phase show a marked tendency to be careless, thoughtless, unpunctual, forgetful, and absent-minded. This inefficiency at a time when they are more likely to try to end their lives may result in a disproportionate failure."

Every suicidal gesture should be taken seriously. A sufferer's mood may deteriorate so suddenly just before or during menstruation that she may attempt suicide at a most unexpected moment. The attempt may end her life, even though it was only intended as a cry for help, or it may result in permanent damage that is even harder to cope with than the premenstrual complaint. Drug overdoses may result in permanent liver or kidney damage, and if a woman throws herself in front of a car or jumps off a bridge, a scarred face or broken limbs will be ever-present reminders of the event that made her life so intolerable. One patient brought in diaries with a record of 40 overdose attempts. Each one had needed hospital admission and had occurred during her premenstruum, those four fateful days before menstruation.

Edith, a 24-year-old executive assistant, wrote:

"On December 6, realizing how dangerous the premenstrual effects were, I felt in great need of help. Unfortunately, my group meeting was during this time, and did not help me at all. After the meeting I rushed home, hid from my boyfriend whom I saw downtown, and intended again to overdose. Luckily, two friends arrived on the scene, and by the time they left it was all over and I had started to menstruate."

When women, particularly young girls, are in deep despair, they may occasionally resort to self-mutilation by slashing their wrists, abdomen, neck or face, or shaving their scalp or eyebrows. They may injure themselves severely, yet they apparently experience no pain and appear to be anesthetized during the process. Self-mutilation is rare in men, and although it can occur in any woman, it appears to be most frequent among sufferers of premenstrual syndrome, so much so that when self-mutilation occurs, it is important to first eliminate the possibility of premenstrual syndrome before resorting to routine antidepressant therapy.

Depression can be an emotional reaction, such as when we hear of the death of a close friend or of other bad news, but it can also be an illness, and affect bodily functions as well. The symptoms of a depressive illness are similar to premenstrual depression, but there are differences, one being the timing. In a depressive illness the symptoms are present day after day throughout the entire month, and may last for weeks, months, or years. In premenstrual depression the symptoms are measured in days and do not last longer than 14 days, for after menstruation the woman is her normal self. Another important difference is the marked irritability that accompanies premenstrual depression. Premenstrual depression increases with age after 26 years and is common among single women.

Depression is best thought of as a disease of "loss," for there is a loss of happiness, interests, and enthusiasm, loss of memory, energy, sleep, and sexual arousal. One feels a loss of security and adequacy, and a loss of the powers of concentration, so that it becomes difficult to read a book or follow a television show. There is a loss of self-control and an inability to make decisions or to control one's tears, behavior, and appetite. There is a loss of insight and an inability to realize, in the case of premenstrual depression, that very shortly the symptoms will pass and there will be a return to normalcy.

TIREDNESS

"What worries me most is that I get so slow and stupid before my periods." This comment by a journalist is echoed by many who find the lethargy, exhaustion, and fatigue so difficult to cope with during the premenstruum. The "I-can't-be-bothered" attitude takes over and disrupts the program for the day, until in the end "everything goes."

Frances, a 32-year-old working mother, hated the tiredness most, and wrote:

> "The worst and most worrying symptom is the feeling of apathy that descends on me. All physical and mental activity becomes a real effort and all I want to do is curl up in a corner away from everyone and all my responsibilities. I find it quite frightening that I cannot think clearly or quickly, and feel mentally dulled. These symptoms get increasingly worse, and a couple of days before a period I feel quite ill. The first day of a period I feel a bit headachy and tired, but then it is like a weight being lifted off me and for 2 weeks or so I feel really fine."

This tiredness may lead to withdrawal and a wish to hide, so aptly described by a secretary as:

> ". . . a total withdrawal from all social contacts and withdrawing into myself. Despite living with friends, I often find myself not wanting to speak unless absolutely necessary, and often only manage one or two sentences."

Again, the tiredness may vary in severity from the typist who fills her wastebasket with typing errors to the executive who feels unable to compose letters and stares all day at a blank sheet of paper. A mother of two boys, aged 1 and 3, wrote:

> "When I feel bad I stay in bed all day. One day during my last vacation I felt so bad I couldn't bear to lift my sons or get them dressed, so the poor kids had to stay in bed the whole day. I just cried and told them how sorry I was that I couldn't help them at all. I'm afraid the little ones who have known me like this may grow up into disturbed children, but I promise you I'm quite normal at other times in my cycle."

One woman, not yet known to me, called for an appointment and when describing her tiredness, added:

> "I seem to be in a daze on those days. I can't do anything right—more than once I've crossed the road to go to the restroom and found myself in the Men's Room."

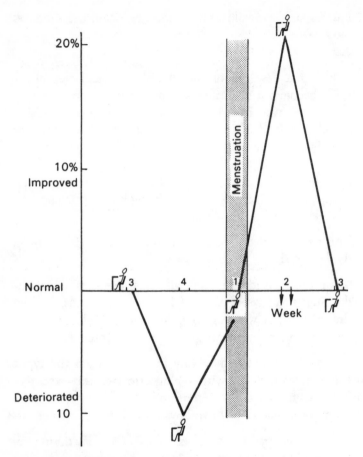

Figure 9   Variation in schoolgirls' weekly grades with
            menstruation

Another patient confessed that:

> "Just before a period, for about 10 days, a sleepiness takes
> me over and all I want to do is sit down and sleep, so that
> no housework or proper cooking gets done."

It is premenstrual fatigue that is responsible for the drop in
mental ability before menstruation. At one girl's boarding school
in the south of England 1,561 weekly grades were studied and
compared with the previous week's grades. Each grade covered

the total scores of some seven to twelve different subjects. During the premenstrual week there was an average drop of 10%, compared with a compensatory rise of 20% during the week immediately following menstruation. (See Figure 9.) This effect is also evident in high school and college level examination results.

IRRITABILITY

Those who are closest to a sufferer of premenstrual irritability are most affected by her short fuse and explosions over trivial matters. This usually includes not only the nearest but also the dearest—the husband or partner, and children, or parents. As one woman said:

> "Pity those around me when the least things upset me. I hate everyone, I shout and pick quarrels, and the whole world gets on my nerves."

Premenstrual irritability is more common in married women. Husbands naturally have problems trying to deal with their supersensitive, edgy, irrational, and agitated wives during these days of each cycle. Too many cases end up with visits to a marriage counselor or in divorce.

The following three excerpts from letters suggest that the husband often suffers as much as his wife:

> "I have been suffering from premenstrual tension for some years now, and recently it came to its height. I was in my usual depressed state and, being angry, didn't know what to do with myself, just lost my temper for the thousandth time and I kicked in the door and required 40 stitches in my leg. My husband is at his wits' end. He doesn't know what to do with me, not knowing what I'm going to do next, and is ready to leave me after being married only 18 months. I keep telling him that I'll be good the next time, but I never am and just can't control myself."

> "Last Saturday I deliberately smashed all the dishes after clearing the table. I started menstruating in the evening.

My family doctor puts it down to my Irish temper. I get so depressed, hateful, and tired; I stay in bed and shout, and I could go on and on like this. It is my husband who asked me to write for help."

"At 32, there is very little hope for me except, perhaps, menopause. I have a history of suicide attempts, child- and husband-beating, and many fights with a long-suffering doctor, who has been accused by me of many crimes, neglect and attempted manslaughter among them. At my worst I have taken many prescribed antidepressants in massive overdoses."

If one sees a patient shortly after an aggressive outburst like those described above, it may be possible to get full details of the time at which food was taken during the day. It is a common finding that the irritability is always worse when, in addition to premenstrual tension, there has been a long interval since the last meal, causing the blood sugar level to fall (see the discussion on blood sugar levels in Chapter 16). When patients are asked at what time of day their irritability increases, it is usually in the late morning if breakfast has been missed, or when preparing the evening meal or waiting for the husband if he is later than usual. Often the wife has only had a sandwich, or just cheese and an apple at midday, and has eaten nothing else in anticipation of the evening meal.

Sudden explosive outbursts of irritability or aggression can usually be helped by ensuring that regular small meals are taken at intervals of 3 hours. In two recent cases of murder and one of infanticide, it was found that no food had been taken for 9 hours.

At the height of the tension there may be true confusion and memory loss, so that the woman is unaware of her actions or surroundings. Indeed, she may bitterly deny her actions, for she has no memory of them. The following notes made by a patient show how extreme the confusion may be, and how it may well represent temporary insanity.

"From the fourth onward, severe depression with secretive confusion. On the seventh I planned to kill my mother and myself. I wrote suicide notes to all concerned and took certain prescribed drugs that I thought would work. I do not know whether I would have done it, as my friend, with whom I have a good relationship, discovered them and flushed them down the toilet. It took quite a few days before I realized how bizarre the whole episode was. The loss of appetite, need for alcohol, aggression, lack of interest, and swollen glands continued until menstruation started on the ninth. These notes are written on the eighteenth when my mind is clear."

It is not surprising that premenstrual tension, with its irritability and confusion, frequently leads to problems with the law. There are those cases of aggression where, in a sudden fit of temper, a woman makes an unjustified assault on her neighbor or boss, or violently attacks a police officer. There are cases of baby-battering, husband-beating, and homicide, mentioned earlier. Becoming drunk and disorderly when under the influence of alcohol or drugs may also lead to charges. In France it is recognized that premenstrual tension may become so acute and so violent that it may be classified as "temporary insanity" in courts of law.

My British survey, in 1961, of 156 newly incarcerated women prisoners revealed that half had committed their crime during the paramenstruum, and that premenstrual syndrome was present in two-thirds of these women who committed their crime during the paramenstruum. Theft was the most common crime, with 56% of incidents committed during the paramenstruum, while the alcoholics charged with being "drunk and disorderly" were a close second at 54%. In the same women's prison 20 years later, two psychiatrists, Dr. D'Orban and Joy Dalton (no relation to the author), confirmed these findings in relation to crimes of violence, finding 44% had committed their offense during the paramenstruum and 34% suffered from premenstrual syndrome.

The Paris police noticed early in this century that 84% of crimes of violence by women had been committed during the premenstruum or menstruation. This was confirmed by a similar study in New York, which showed that 62% of crimes of violence occurred during the premenstruum.

Dr. Morton and his colleagues, working in Westfield State Prison, Bedford Hills, New York, showed that it was worthwhile treating the inmates of prisons and reformatories if they suffered from premenstrual syndrome. He found that treatment resulted in an increased work output, less punishment for disobeying rules, and an increase in general morale.

In fact, the question should be asked: What benefit will a woman gain from a prison sentence or fine if she is unable to control her premenstrual irritability or confusion? Most premenstrual syndrome prisoners, if untreated, usually serve their full sentences without remission for good conduct, because their symptoms get the better of them each premenstruum and cause further problems.

5

Waterlogged

For some women the days from ovulation to menstruation are characterized by bloatedness, heaviness, and/or a gain in weight. The sensation of bloatedness is caused by the fluid outside the cells seeping into and expanding individual cells, and it does not necessarily mean that there is a gain in weight. The weight-gain may be due to an accumulation of water in the tissues and cells of the body, because only part of the water that is taken in during those two weeks is being passed out, while some remains and gradually accumulates. In addition to water, sodium may also be retained while potassium may be lost. It should be stressed that water-retention is only one of the many symptoms of premenstrual syndrome, and many women never experience it at all, even though they may suffer from severe premenstrual syndrome.

The most common sign of water being retained in the body is an increase in weight, which generally averages 4–7 pounds (see Figure 10) but can be even more, as much as 10–12 pounds. The normal weight is that which is taken during the postmenstruum, and gains and losses of up to 3 pounds are usually considered within normal limits for women. Dr. William Thomas of Chicago documented a case of one woman who gained between 12 and 14 pounds each premenstruum, and then lost it with an excessive output of 9 pints of urine on the first

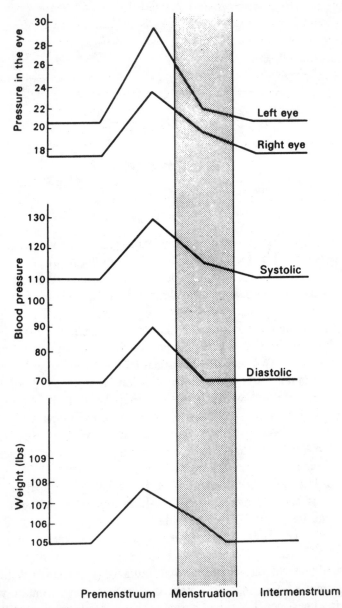

Figure 10 Fluctuations during the menstrual cycle in weight,
blood pressure, and pressure in the eye of a sufferer
of premenstrual syndrome

day of menstruation, the excessive urine output continuing for the next few days. Those who regularly gain and lose very large amounts of water periodically are sometimes diagnosed as suffering from "cyclical idiopathic edema."

Early workers on premenstrual syndrome believed that the amount of premenstrual weight gain was an index of the severity of premenstrual symptoms, but this is definitely not the case. Dr. Bruce and Professor Russell of Maudsley Hospital, London, examined 34 women who complained of premenstrual symptoms. They carefully measured their weights and the amount of fluids they took in and the amount they passed out, and found no relationship. In fact, they wrongly concluded from this that premenstrual syndrome was a purely psychological condition.

Apart from the gain in weight, water retention shows itself in the different tissues, with varying effects, as experienced by *Gladys* who wrote:

> "The pattern of a 5-pound weight increase at period times makes me so bloated that I no longer fit in my favorite slacks, and I feel ready to burst. My breasts become enlarged and sore, needing a larger size bra, my eyes get sunken, and I get dark rings under them. There is extreme fatigue, both physical, so that I can hardly put one foot before the other, and mental, so that I feel incapable of dealing with the children I teach. I get into black depressions, caused by trivial things going wrong. I get throbbing and severe headaches in the week before my period, and always during the first 3 days of bleeding. I work a full-time job, look after the home and three children, and go to evening classes. I also paint and do flower arranging . . . so you see I do try to fight it."

BREAST SORENESS

Complaints of breast soreness with enlarged and tender nipples are common in PMS. Frequently, this leads to fears that this may be a sign of cancer of the breast. It is definitely not related to cancer in any way. What is happening is that the breast tissue is getting ready in the event that, following ovulation, a pregnancy will occur, and the breasts will be needed for breast-feeding. It must be emphasized that not all cases of breast tenderness are because of premenstrual syndrome; only those cases where cyclical soreness is present in the premenstruum with complete absence of pain after menstruation. Breast swelling that is present throughout the month but more marked in the paramenstruum may be caused by increased output of the hormone prolactin from the pituitary gland. It is possible to measure the blood prolactin level, and if this is high, treatment with bromocriptine may help. It must not be forgotten that breasts are sexually charged areas, and when a woman is having problems in her sex life, her breasts may become more sensitive. Nipple sensitivity, as opposed to breast tenderness, may also result from taking vitamin B-6, even low dosages, over a long period. (See pages 212–214.)

FLUID RETENTION

The extra water in the tissues can cause ankles and fingers to swell, so that shoes have to be discarded and rings removed. There may be swelling of the gums, so that dentures no longer fit. The skin coarsens and becomes blotchy, contact lenses won't fit, and the hair becomes stringy. One model, who refused to accept work during the premenstruum, said:

> "I look my very worst—my skin won't take make-up, my face goes stiff, and I can't move gracefully with those extra pounds of weight!"

The exact place where the water accumulates varies in different women and at different times in their life. The most severe symptoms result from water accumulating in a small un-stretchable area such as the labyrinth of the inner ear, which causes dizziness; when it enters the eyeball, causing raised pressure inside the eye and severe pain; and when it occurs inside the unyielding, bony skull, causing headaches. The sinuses are air spaces within the bones of the face where air enters through a small entrance that is lined with cells of the mucus membrane. When these are engorged and swollen, the entrance to the sinus is blocked, causing stale air to accumulate and resulting in sinus headaches or "vacuum headaches." Water can also accumulate in the discs between the vertebrae of the spine, causing backaches.

Sometimes there is a widespread distribution of the extra water, which produces vague symptoms in the muscles, joints, and soft tissues, causing generalized rheumatic pains, abdominal bloating, and heaviness. The water is always in the cells or in the fluid between the cells, it is never free, although one patient imagined she could hear the water "splashing inside her abdomen," and another described how her abdomen was "gurgling and swimming in water." When the extra water accumulates in the fat and subcutaneous tissues, there can be an appreciable gain in weight, without any other complaints. This is most likely to happen in obese women. One speaker at a medical lecture observed, tongue-in-cheek, that "Today, no woman suffers from obesity, only from water retention."

LOCATING THE WATER

The actual sites where the cells become swollen may vary from time to time, depending on factors such as (1) anatomical abnormality, (2) heredity, (3) injury, and (4) infection. Thus, a premenstrual sinus headache is more likely to occur in a woman whose nose cartilage is bent. Water is readily attracted to cells that have recently been injured or infected, so that after a fracture of the leg or arm it is usual to notice premenstrual swelling there for some months. If water retention occurs during the premenstruum in someone who has recently had pneumonia, it may cause a return of the cough or breathlessness.

This water retention is often blamed for the depression and other symptoms that accompany it. Helen, a 27-year-old accountant, wrote:

> "I start to get tender, swollen breasts, usually 14 days (ovulation?) before the beginning of menstruation, and I gain several pounds in weight. This makes me depressed and bad-tempered, and when you feel like that you can't help getting annoyed with everyone around you."

Many of the symptoms of water retention are typically worse in the early morning, often waking the patient from her sleep. This is especially so with migraines, with the acute pain in the eyeball that mimics glaucoma, and with asthma, when there is swelling of the lining cells of the small tubes of the lung. Some people are awakened by a feeling of pins and needles, and perhaps numbness of their fingers. This is because the nerve passes from the arm through a narrow bony tunnel at the wrist, and when the surrounding cells are swollen and waterlogged, this nerve becomes constricted. This odd sensation is called "carpal tunnel syndrome."

Many drugs are available nowadays that help to increase the amount of urine passed, and these would seem to be a simple answer to the problem of water retention. Unfortunately, the problem is not quite so simple. Although these drugs or diuretics can get rid of water, extra water forms again, quickly. It is rather like bailing water from a boat with a hole in it: it is better to close up the hole and prevent further water entering than to just keep bailing. And as bailers get tired, so do the water tablets. The temptation then is to use stronger and stronger drugs to get rid of more and more water. But, as mentioned earlier, the problem is not only that water accumulates, but that potassium is also lost. Diuretics cause water and more potassium to pass in the urine, so unless sufficient potassium is added there may be a marked lowering of the blood potassium level, resulting in increased tiredness and possibly also weakness of the legs. Doctors can estimate the blood potassium level to know how much potassium is circulating in the blood at a given moment, but this does not indicate how much potassium is actually present in the cells, or in the fluid between the cells, which is what really matters. There is now a new class of potassium-sparing diuretics that do not upset the potassium level, and these should be the first choice if diuretics are really needed in premenstrual syndrome.

Patients who have received diuretics continually for many years become dehydrated. If the diuretics are stopped suddenly, these patients complain strongly, within a day or two, of feeling bloated. They need to be persuaded to gradually taper off their diuretics, using them every other day, starting immediately after menstruation. After a month or two it may be possible to decrease the dose to every third or fourth day, until they are only used when the weight gain is really marked.

When a woman starts to gain weight, there is the very natural temptation to start dieting. This can be beneficial if her weight is above the ideal for her age and height, but she needs to be careful which diet she chooses. A diet of only fruit juice and liquids will not work, as this will merely increase the water retention. If she tries to solve the problem by missing meals, she risks the possibility of her blood sugar level dropping abnormally low, thus increasing the depression and irritability. Dr. Jerome W. Conn of Michigan was the first to describe, in 1955, a condition of primary aldosteronism, known as Conn's syndrome. He probably knows more than anyone about water, salt, and potassium balance, and he has suggested that the body's reaction to a low blood sugar level is also related to the amount of potassium in the cells. He has shown that the blood sugar level can be improved by correcting the potassium deficiency that may be present. (See Chapter 16.)

Another problem is that water retention does not *cause* premenstrual tension, depression, tiredness, or irritability, so none of these symptoms will be relieved by diuretics. Actually, diuretics are useful only in the short term until progesterone treatment can be given, or in mild cases where they can be used sparingly with the addition of extra potassium if blood tests show this is needed.

6

Monthly Headaches

Many women, looking for a good reason, might be tempted to claim that their particular variety of headache only comes at period time. Undoubtedly, menstruation is the most frequent time for migraine attacks in women. This is shown in Figure 11, in which the times of 935 migraine attacks are shown in relation to the days of the menstrual cycle. On the other hand, those who can produce a 3-month record showing a regular and definite relationship of their headache to menstruation have a much better chance of obtaining relief through progesterone treatment. In Figure 12 we can see that Isobel's headaches last between 7 and 10 days before each period, and are preceded by symptoms of tension, which ease off during menstruation. Joan presents a different picture: her headaches last only 1 or 2 days, and there is no premenstrual tension, but the headaches all tend to come around the time of menstruation. Kathleen seems to have headaches every 10 or 12 days; occasionally they coincide with menstruation, but often they just come at any time. It is unlikely that Kathleen will benefit from hormonal treatment.

Generally, the monthly headaches that are likely to benefit from treatment with specific hormones such as progesterone are those that show a definite relationship to menstruation in a 3-month record, and those headaches that started either at puberty, after a pregnancy, or while on the pill. These women are likely to be free from headaches after the fourth month of pregnancy, and may well look back to the later months of pregnancy as the only time in their life when they knew what that freedom was like. Unfortunately, these same women are also likely to say that immediately after their pregnancy the headaches returned worse than ever.

Women who find their headaches becoming worse while they are on the pill or who have a tendency to headaches on the first or second day after stopping the course of pills, are likely to be responsive to hormone treatment. The majority of

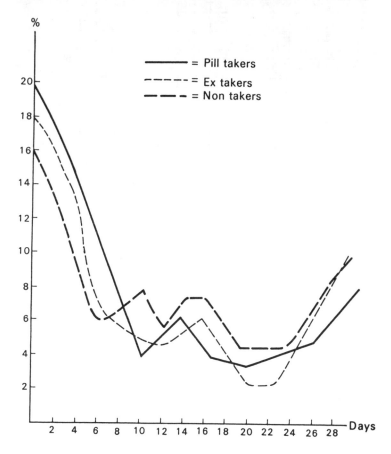

Figure 11 935 migraine attacks in relation to the menstrual cycle

	Isobel				Joan				Kathleen			
	Jan.	Feb.	Mar.	Apr.	May.	Jun.	Jul.	Aug.	Sep.	Oct.	Nov.	Dec.
1	hT	hT	M									M
2	hT	HT	M						H			
3	hT	HT	M								M	
4	nT	HM									M	
5	HT	M									M	
6	HT	M						H			M	H
7	HT	M		T				M		H		
8	HM	M		T				M				
9	nM			T			H	M				
10	hM			T	H			M				
11	M		T	Th	H	H	M	M		M	H	
12	M		T	Th	M	Mh	M			M		
13	M		T	Th	M	M	M			M		
14			Th	Th	M	M	M		M			
15			Th	Th	M	M	M		M			
16			Th	TH	M	M			M			
17			Th	TH		M						
18		T	Th	M								
19		T	TH	M								
20		T	TH	M								
21		Th	H	M								
22	T	Th	HM						H	H		
23	T	Th	HM									
24	T	HT	M									M
25	nT	HM	M									M
26	hT	hM	M									M
27	hT	M										
28	hT	M										
29	hT										M	
30	hT								H		M	
31	hT											
Total												

h = Mild headache   M = Menstruation

H = Severe headache   T = Tension

Figure 12 Headaches in relation to menstruation

these women are also likely to find that after menopause most of their problems come to an end.

The three common types of headaches related to menstruation are (1) sinus or vacuum headaches, (2) tension headaches, and (3) migraines.

VACUUM HEADACHES

It is better to speak of "vacuum headaches" rather than "sinus headaches," as the latter are likely to be confused with the headaches resulting from true sinusitis, which is caused by infected material getting lodged in the sinuses, and are not likely to be related to menstruation. Vacuum headaches, on the other

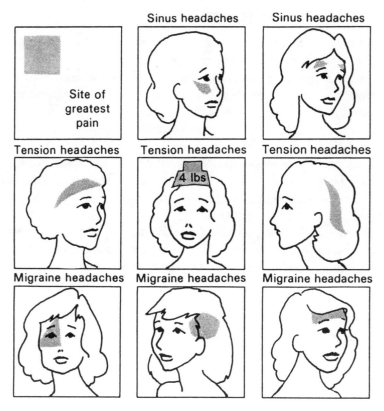

Figure 13 Sites of greatest pain in menstrual headaches

hand, are caused by the swelling of the cells at the entrance to the sinus, which block the entry so that stale air accumulates inside. Women generally know that a headache is on the way when their nasal passages become blocked and it is difficult to breathe through one nostril. There is tenderness or pressure over the sinuses, which are situated in the cheekbones and over the eyes. The pain that results is made worse by bending over, and may last from 1–7 days. In addition, there may be other signs of waterlogging, such as a gain in weight, bloated abdomen, shortness of breath, or swollen ankles or fingers. These women would be wise to restrict their fluid intake to 4 cups of liquid daily, and may benefit from nasal decongestants.

TENSION HEADACHES

Tension headaches usually have a slow onset, so that a woman who is trying to chart her symptoms may be uncertain whether the pain in her head is bad enough to call a headache. A tension headache usually starts after symptoms of premenstrual tension—irritability, tiredness, or depression—and eases off gradually during the course of menstruation. The pain from tension headaches has been described as "a steel band enclosing my head," or "like a heavy weight on top of my head." (See Figure 13.) These women will find that the usual analgesics such as aspirin or paracetamol will only give relief for about 4 hours, then the headache returns and the analgesic must be repeated. Treatment with progesterone (see Chapter 21) is most valuable for this type of headache, and it has the added advantage of relieving the other symptoms of premenstrual syndrome.

MIGRAINES

Doctors like to divide migraines into two varieties: the classical and the common. In the classical variety the patient has a warning or "aura" that lasts for about 20 minutes before the onset of a severe headache. This aura may be sudden flashes of lights, brightly colored stars and stripes, or a patch of blindness; or there may be a sensation of pins and needles in the tongue, the side of the face, or the hands and legs. Many people suffer both classical and common migraine at different times over the years. Common migraine has no aura and begins gradually, increasing in severity. Both migraines may be accompanied by nausea or vomiting and extreme fatigue, and usually last between 24 and 48 hours, although some unlucky women find they last even longer.

Most migraine sufferers have a family history, with a parent, brothers, sisters, uncles, or aunts also suffering, so they start life with a predisposition to migraines. Nevertheless, there are those among them whose attacks are related to menstruation and can benefit from simple advice and possibly also from progesterone treatment.

In order to help women who have frequent or severe migraine attacks, it is helpful to have full details of all they have been doing, and of the times at which any food has been consumed. In practice, an attack form like that shown in Figure 14 proves valuable, and helps to isolate an individual trigger factor. The trigger factor is the last straw, which decides exactly when a migraine is going to occur in a susceptible woman. It is often the result of either going too long without food, so that there is a drop in the blood sugar level, or of eating foods to which the sufferer is sensitive.

Name............................   Date...............................
                                 Day of week.......................
                                 Time of onset ....
                                 Duration ....
Day of cycle......................   Days before next menstruation......

During the 24 hours *before* an attack:—

(1) Did you have any special worry, overwork or shock?
(2) What had you done during the day?
        Normal work?
        Unusual activity?
        Extra tired?
(3) What food had you eaten and when?
        Breakfast.....................   Time...........................
        ....
        Mid-morning..................   Time...........................
        ....
        Lunch........................   Time...........................
        ....
        Mid-afternoon.................   Time...........................
        ....
        Supper ....   Time...........................
        ....
        Evening ....   Time...........................
        ....
        Bedtime ....   Time...........................
        ....

Figure 14 An attack form useful for isolating trigger factors in migraine

TOO LONG WITHOUT FOOD

When women are asked what sort of things start a migraine attack, they often mention travel, theater-going, or working hard for several days for a special event, like a garage sale, a wedding, or a big party. If the attack forms have been carefully filled in, it is usually easy to spot if the migraine has been caused by too long an interval without food. Generally speaking, 5 hours between meals is long enough for most women leading a normal energetic life. Women with premenstrual syndrome will find that over 3 hours without food (see pages 149–152) can be too long an interval. An overnight interval of 13 hours is usually considered the limit. After this length of time susceptible women, probably those already born with the tendency to get migraines, will find they develop a headache. This explains why travel often causes a headache: with frequent interruptions and long distances traveled, meals are often delayed longer than usual. Similarly, if one is busy with preparations for special events, food may easily be forgotten. And if you are giving the party, how easy it is to ensure that your guests have plenty while you forget to eat anything yourself.

One must also consider not only the interval between meals, but the amount of energy expended during the interval. The more energy is used, the quicker the blood sugar level falls. Overnight fasting is often the cause of a migraine attack on waking, and there are those migraine sufferers who say they cannot sleep late on holidays or on the weekend because they wake up with a headache. Migraines are also likely to occur when the evening meal is followed by some energetic sport or a brisk walk and no further food is taken before going to bed.

An example of this was noted in a receptionist who was an avid skater and normally had her evening meal at 6:30 P.M. On Thursday evenings she would go to the rink for 3 hours of energetic recreation, but would have no food after the evening meal. Every 4 or 5 weeks, she would wake with a migraine on Friday mornings. The attacks occurred during the paramenstruum, but were triggered off by the long interval without food and the energetic skating.

Full information about the effect of a drop in blood sugar levels is given on pages 149–152. If the attack forms show that the woman has gone without food for too long or has been too energetic for the amount of food she has had, a sudden drop in blood sugar may have triggered the attack. In that case the treatment is obvious: avoid fasting, and remember to have an extra cookie with your morning and afternoon coffee or tea. Remember, too, that proteins such as meat, fish, and eggs will keep the blood sugar up longer, while candy will cause a short, sharp rise in blood sugar level followed by a quick drop, and thus provide only a temporary benefit.

FOODS CAUSING MIGRAINES

Women whose migraine attacks are not caused by fasting may find that they are sensitive to certain foods, the most common of which are cheese, chocolate, alcohol, and citrus fruits. A few are sensitive to ripe bananas, pork, onions, fish, and gluten. In these cases the migraine attacks do not occur immediately after the specific food has been eaten, but some 12–36 hours later. This is because the attack occurs not when the food is digested in the stomach, but later, when it is broken down in the liver by the action of the special chemicals known as "enzymes." Apparently, if one particular enzyme is not present, a wrong chemical action occurs, releasing substances capable of opening wide the blood vessels of the brain. These substances are known as vasodilating amines. Two common ones are tyramine, which is present in cheese, and phenylethylamine, which is present in alcohol and chocolate; but there are many other vasodilating amines that can be formed by the wrong breakdown of everyday foods. Some women's sensitivity to vasodilating amines may be increased during the paramenstruum, so that although they are able to take small amounts of, say, cheese, after menstruation, as menstruation approaches, or during menstruation, even a minute amount is sufficient to provoke an attack.

Women who fall into this category should try to avoid the foods to which they are sensitive, remembering always that it is an individual problem. Foods that cause attacks in one individ-

ual will not necessarily cause attacks in another migraine sufferer. However, as mentioned earlier, there are often other members of the family who also suffer from migraines, so it may be
worthwhile having a "gathering of the clan" at which all blood
relations who suffer from migraine can exchange ideas. Often,
they may find a common food to which all family members are
sensitive.

Those who are sensitive to cheese will be happy to learn
that tyramine is not present in cream or cottage cheese, but
only develops on maturing, so among the particular cheeses to
be avoided are Stilton, Cheddar, parmesan, and processed cheeses.
However, they should be aware that mature cheese is often
hidden in quiches, Mornay sauce, and Italian dishes.

Red wine, sherry, port, and champagne are probably the
worst alcohols for causing migraines, but it is often possible to
take a single glass of white wine with food without any aftereffects. It is also worth considering the difference between grape
and grain alcohols, for more people are sensitive to grape alcohols than to grain alcohols like beer, vodka, and whiskey.

Chocolate is often added to rich fruit cakes or finger cakes
to give a good color, and to coffee dishes to increase the flavor,
so those who are sensitive to chocolate should be on their
guard. Plain dark chocolate is more likely to provoke an attack
than mild chocolate. And how easy it is for those sensitive to
citrus fruits to forget that this also includes mandarins and
tangerines.

7

❧

Recurrent Problems

My interest in premenstrual syndrome was first aroused within a few days of qualifying as a doctor while I was working as a fill-in for a general practitioner. In the early hours of the morning I received a call from a 34-year-old mother of three children, who had an acute attack of asthma. The husband, who opened the door, was most apologetic for calling at such an hour, but added, "Unfortunately it happens every month, except when she's pregnant."

The woman certainly had a severe asthmatic attack, and I quickly gave her an injection to ease her breathing. As I was driving home, the husband's words reminded me of my own migraine, which also occurred once a month, just before menstruation. I recalled that the only times of freedom for me, too, had been during my pregnancies. A visit to the patient later that day revealed that her first attack of asthma had occurred at the age of 17, coinciding with her first period, and she had had an attack of asthma with each menstruation thereafter. The medical textbooks did not mention this possibility, but Dr. Raymond Greene, who had helped me with my migraine, suggested that this patient should also be treated with progesterone. In those days only doctors could give injections, and during that first month, while giving the asthma patient her daily injections, I came across another woman with premenstrual asthma, two with premenstrual epilepsy, and one with premenstrual migraine. So did the story of the premenstrual syndrome begin.

In the early years it was essentially the physical ailments that were noticed, with much less appreciation of tension and other psychological symptoms. A survey in 1982 of 1,095 women who were being treated with progesterone for premenstrual syndrome, compared with the symptoms reported in the first article in the *British Medical Journal* in 1953, emphasizes the differences:

	1953	1982
Headache	69%	33%
Depression	6%	35%
Vertigo	13%	3%
Skin lesions	13%	3%
Bloatedness	6%	31%
Asthma	5%	1%
Epilepsy	5%	1%
Breast tenderness	2%	21%

The only way to identify a chronic recurring symptom as being part of premenstrual syndrome is to chart it carefully, together with the days of menstruation, for at least three months. If this was done more frequently, there would be many more women whose asthma, epilepsy, migraines, and numerous other complaints would be identified as menstrually related. At present, the list of symptoms that can be related to premenstrual syndrome is almost endless and certainly covers all the systems of the body. This means that almost all specialists, no matter what their discipline, are likely to encounter its effects. In fact, many of these symptoms are among the most common that the specialist is called upon to treat. For instance, the neurologist sees most patients with headaches and epilepsy, the dermatologist sees many patients with acne and boils, the urologist sees patients with cystitis and urethritis, and so on.

Women with bodily, or somatic, symptoms related to menstruation will have the usual characteristics of premenstrual syndrome. They will have the onset at puberty, after pregnancy or use of the pill, or when menstruation resumes after a few months absence. They will be free from symptoms in later pregnancy, and their symptoms will be eased after menopause. There will be a high number whose symptoms start after a pregnancy complicated by pre-eclamptic toxemia, postnatal depression, or sterilization.

While it is impractical to list all the possible symptoms of premenstrual syndrome, the common ones are discussed below. (See Figure 15.)

Premenstrual asthma appears to be caused by water retention in the cells lining the smaller tubes of the lung, which become swollen and prevent the free entry of air into the minute air sacs. Thus the cause is not necessarily allergic. In fact, these patients may not respond to sodium cromoglycate (Intal) inhalers, as do those whose asthma has a definite allergic basis. Premenstrual asthma is particularly common in women in their thirties and forties. Usually, the women will say that their attacks are brought on by tension and stress, but that may be because they have not yet related them to premenstrual tension. In the special asthma clinics in hospitals it is usual for about one-third of all women of childbearing age to have menstrually related asthma. Two women, aged 18 and 42, who were treated at the PMS Clinic at the University College Hospital, London, had a record of over 20 admissions to intensive care units for acute asthma. Finally, an alert nurse noticed that their attacks always occurred premenstrually. Both have since become free from asthma after receiving progesterone treatment.

One of the most satisfying experiences for a doctor is to be able to diagnose and treat a woman with **premenstrual epilepsy.** She can be treated with progesterone, and taken off all anticonvulsant tablets, with their many unpleasant side effects. Furthermore, in Britain, if a person is not taking anti-convulsant drugs and has been 3 years without an epileptic fit, she has the joy of having her driver's license restored.

Premenstrual epilepsy is often a culminating symptom,

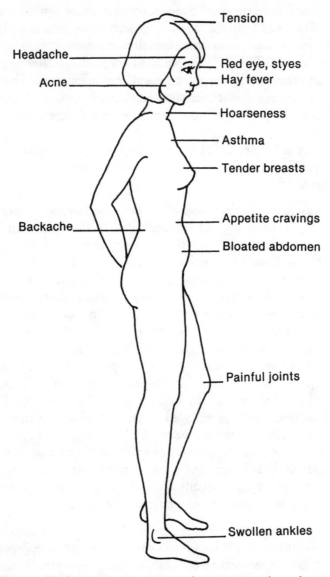

Figure 15 Common symptoms of premenstrual syndrome

which follows gradually increasing tension and headache, so these patients do have a warning that an attack is imminent. There may also be marked weight-gain, though this is not al-

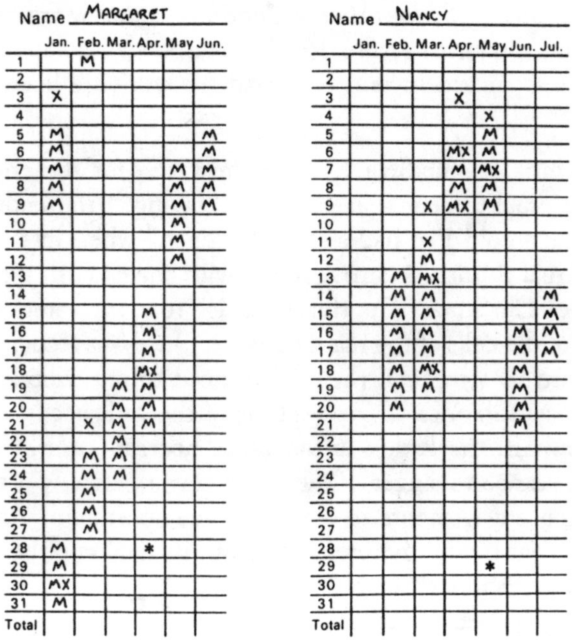

Name **MARGARET**

	Jan.	Feb.	Mar.	Apr.	May	Jun.
1		M				
2						
3	X					
4						
5	M					M
6	M					M
7	M				M	M
8	M				M	M
9	M				M	M
10					M	
11					M	
12					M	
13						
14						
15				M		
16				M		
17				M		
18				MX		
19			M	M		
20			M	M		
21		X	M	M		
22			M			
23		M	M			
24		M	M			
25		M				
26		M				
27		M				
28	M			*		
29	M					
30	MX					
31	M					
Total						

Margaret is 27 yrs old with 2 children, onset after 1st pregnancy

Name **NANCY**

	Jan.	Feb.	Mar.	Apr.	May	Jun.	Jul.
1							
2							
3				X			
4					X		
5					M		
6				MX	M		
7				M	MX		
8				M	M		
9			X	MX	M		
10							
11			X				
12			M				
13		M	MX				
14		M	M				M
15		M	M				M
16		M	M			M	M
17		M	M			M	M
18		M	MX			M	
19		M	M			M	
20		M				M	
21						M	
22							
23							
24							
25							
26							
27							
28							
29					*		
30							
31							
Total							

Nancy is 28 yrs old, onset at puberty

M = menstruation
X = epileptic attack
* = progesterone treatment started

Figure 16 Charts of two patients with premenstrual epilepsy

ways the case. Often the final trigger factor that precipitates the attack is a long interval without food.

Laura, 28 years old, with one child, left for her vacation having had only a light breakfast at 8 A.M. Her husband drove some 300 miles, stopping only to ask the way. When she arrived at her hotel she had a nasty headache, and while she was unpacking, at about 5 P.M., she had an epileptic fit. She started menstruating the next day. She later agreed that there had been mounting tension during the previous week, which she had attributed to trying to finish all the necessary jobs in time for her vacation.

The charts of two other epileptic patients, Margaret and Nancy, are shown in Figure 16. Both responded completely to progesterone treatment and both had their driver's licenses restored.

Rhinitis or Hayfever is often mistaken for the **common cold.** It is usual to hear women in April saying, " You know, this is the fourth cold I've had since Christmas," when in fact it is premenstrual rhinitis occurring along with their fourth menstruation since Christmas. The rhinitis is due to extra water causing swelling of the cells of the nasal passages. Once it is recognized as a premenstrual symptom, there is no need to prescribe antihistamines or antibiotics. If the swelling of the cells occurs a little lower down in the larynx it can cause **hoarseness,** which is a special nuisance to singers. One opera singer carefully arranged her singing engagements to avoid her premenstruum. Another remarked that during the premenstruum the quality of her voice changed, and she was unable to reach the high notes. This was corrected by progesterone therapy.

The **loss of a sense of smell** is probably more common than generally appreciated. It is caused by extra water accumulating in the cells that are responsible for the sense of smell. The manufacturer of a special brand of antiperspirant/deodorant noticed that women tended to change their brand every 3 or 4 weeks, complaining that it had ceased to function effectively. Market research showed that the dissatisfaction was due to a premenstrual increase in perspiration and vaginal discharge, and a diminishing ability to smell the reassuring perfume of the antiperspirant/ deodorant product. This led women to believe that the product had lost its effectiveness.

Dizziness or **vertigo** is a common premenstrual complaint. In some surveys it occurred in one-third of all sufferers of premenstrual syndrome. It is most frequent among those who have had children and are approaching menopause. The dizziness gets worse if the woman bends over, and it may accompany a headache. The probable cause is excess fluid in the labyrinth of the ear, which is responsible for balance.

Similarly, **fainting** is common just before menstruation, and is most likely to occur when there has been a long interval without food, or prolonged standing. In England it is common among teenage schoolgirls who have missed their breakfast and have to stand for a long time at the early morning school assembly.

Cystitis and **urethritis** are common symptoms during the premenstruum, and may be caused by the increase in vaginal discharge and generalized pelvic congestion.

Joint and **muscle pains** may come back each month just before menstruation, last only a few days, and then disappear without treatment. There may also be stiffness on waking in the morning, although this disappears within the hour. The pain is probably caused by localized swelling of the cells, or failure of muscle relaxation during the time of premenstrual tension. The water retention that accompanies many of these symptoms led to the mistaken theory that premenstrual syndrome was due to water retention, and could therefore be corrected by diuretics. The effect of such treatment has already been discussed.

There are many factors responsible for the formation of **varicose veins,** including a tendency within the family. However, when they first begin to appear they may only be visible in the premenstruum, and later they may be painful only at this time of the cycle.

Boils, sties, and **acne** are all common skin lesions, which frequently recur each cycle just before menstruation. Acne is perhaps a special case. It is caused by the grease (or sebum) produced by the sebaceous glands in the skin being too thick and plentiful. This grease is excreted through the pores of the skin. If the grease is too thick, it blocks the pores and causes acne. The skin only starts making grease, or sebum, at puberty, so in the first few years of its production there is often either too much, or it is too thick or too thin. Gradually, the body learns to make the right amount. Estrogen helps to slow down the production of grease, so acne often returns at the time of falling estrogen levels, such as at ovulation and before menstruation. This also explains why acne usually improves during pregnancy when there is plenty of estrogen, and also in some women on the high dosage estrogen pill.

Conjunctivitis, or red eye, may return each month due to causes other than infection. It is interesting that the association of conjunctivitis and menstruation was known as long ago as the sixteenth century.

Glaucoma is caused by raised pressure within the eyeball. This may be due to a narrowing of the opening through which the circulating fluid in the eyeball drains. It is not surprising to find that when there is water retention during the premenstruum, there may be an excess accumulation of fluid within the eye, and also difficulty in draining it away. (See Figure 10.) When this happens the pressure within the eye is raised, which becomes very painful and, by pressure on the optic nerve, may interfere with the sight. A survey of patients of menstruating age with closed-angle glaucoma (where the draining opening is blocked) at the Institute of Ophthalmology, London, revealed that 89% suffered from premenstrual syndrome. **Uveitis** and **iritis** are two other troublesome eye conditions that tend to flare up premenstrually, and respond to progesterone treatment.

Capricious appetite, food cravings, and **binges** are well-known to occur at the height of premenstrual tension and water retention. However great her self-control may be during the rest of the month, there come those days when a woman is just "overtaken by a demon and eats enough for a week in one meal," or "eats like a pig, gorging on sweets."
Olive wrote:

> "My life swings between cycles of feasting and fasting. Having lived on a careful diet of only 750 calories for 2 weeks and losing 4 pounds, I had an uncontrollable urge, which got me out of bed. I raided Mother's pantry and ate two loaves of bread with peanut butter, a packet of ginger cookies, and some apple pie."

Drs. Smith and Sauder from McMaster University, Canada, studied 300 nurses and confirmed that the craving for food and sweets and the desire to eat compulsively occurred during the times of premenstrual depression.

The actual foods chosen when there is compulsive eating are invariably carbohydrates and sweets, suggesting that the body's natural defense is coming into action to prevent a too severe or prolonged drop in blood sugar level. (See Chapter 16.)

Alcoholic binges may be a feature of the paramenstruum. A survey of American female alcoholics revealed that 67% related their drinking to the menstrual cycle. They all felt that their drinking habits had either started or increased during the premenstruum, but that they were able to abstain at other times. During the paramenstruum the process of breaking down the alcohol, which is dependent on an enzyme action in the liver, appears to be slowed, so that more alcohol accumulates in the bloodstream. Many women find they cannot hold their normal amount of alcohol at this time, which is unfortunate, as it implies that care is needed when using alcohol to relieve depression and tension.

Dentists recognize that **ulcers in the mouth** commonly recur during the premenstruum, and these are sometimes accompanied by **ulcers in the vulva, vagina,** and **anus.**

Most opticians have learned that when making appointments for fitting **contact lenses,** they must consider the time of the client's cycle; fitting may prove troublesome during the premenstruum. Similarly, hairdressers know that if a **perm** hasn't taken, the chances are that it was done on the wrong day of the month.

Drug reactions are often reported during the premenstruum, and it is always difficult to know if they were caused by the drug or are a symptom of the premenstruum. This can also produce confusion when doctors are doing controlled tests of new drugs. Often one finds the dummy tablet is effective, whereas the real drug causes headaches, increased drowsiness, or nausea. This may be because the dummy tablet is being taken during the postmenstrual week when the woman is feeling well and the real tablet taken during the premenstruum when she is just reporting her normal premenstrual symptoms.

Mention should also be made of the pain known as **Mittelschmerz,** or "middle pain," which may occur at the time of ovulation. This is usually a mild, cramping pain in the lower abdomen, on one side or the other, usually alternating month by month. It accompanies the release of the egg cell from the ovary, and is possibly caused by the contractions of the tubes as the egg cell makes its way down to the womb. The pain lasts only a few hours, and may be accompanied by a vaginal discharge or even slight bleeding. Young girls are apt to mistake it for acute appendicitis, and more than one teenager has arrived at my office packed and ready to be sent straight off to the hospital. In fact, there is no vomiting, no distention of the abdomen, and none of the usual signs of guarding and localization of pain that doctors normally look for when they examine an abdomen. It is important to have these girls record the time of abdominal pain as well as the dates of menstruation so that they themselves can appreciate the relationship.

Although ovulation occurs alternately on the right and left side, it is not completely regular. For instance, it may be right, right, left, right, left, left. . . so that at the end of the year it will probably have occurred an equal number of times on both sides. This pain, or sensation, should be regarded as Nature's signal that ovulation is occurring, indicating a favorable time for intercourse for those seeking to conceive, or a time for abstinence for those wishing to avoid a pregnancy.

8

Pain and Periods

A very welcome and much needed breeze of common sense wafted through the medical and gynecological fields when Drs. Jean and John Lennane, a husband-and-wife team, pointed out in a well-reasoned paper on a group of disorders including period pain that there is no justification for the old idea that "it is all in the mind." Indeed, all existing scientific evidence points toward a hormonal imbalance being the cause. The Lennanes cite a number of examples from current medical textbooks, which they suggest have led to an irrational and ineffective approach to the treatment of such disorders. These examples included the following:

> "It is generally acknowledged that this condition is much more frequent in the 'highly strung,' nervous, or neurotic female than in her more stable sister."

> "Faulty outlook ... leading to an exaggeration of minor discomfort ... may even be an excuse for not doing something that is disliked."

> "The pain is always secondary to an emotional problem."

> "Very little can be done for a patient who prefers to use menstrual symptoms as a monthly refuge from responsibility and effort."

The idea that period pains, or dysmenorrhea, are purely psychological became widely accepted because there were no abnormalities that could be detected by a physical or gynecological examination, nor are there any suitable tests of hormone levels that can distinguish those who suffer once a month. However, it is gradually being accepted that dysmenorrhea is caused by an imbalance of hormones.

There are two quite different, and in fact opposite, types of dysmenorrhea. One is not premenstrual syndrome, the other is. They are rarely differentiated by the general public, but their treatment is quite different, so it is essential to distinguish between them. There is *spasmodic dysmenorrhea*, characterized by spasms of abdominal pain, which is not premenstrual syndrome, because there is an absence of symptoms in the premenstruum. The other type is *congestive dysmenorrhea*, in which there is increasing congestion, pain, and other symptoms during the premenstruum. Congestive dysmenorrhea has all the characteristics of premenstrual syndrome, in addition to period pains, and so is really premenstrual syndrome. The differences between the two types are clearly shown in the table on the following page.

Spasmodic Dysmenorrhea

When menstruation first starts at puberty no ovulation occurs, nor is there any period pain. About two years later, however, ovulation commences, and then spasmodic dysmenorrhea may also begin. Often, at the beginning, ovulation does not occur every month but only on alternate months, so period pains only occur on alternate months. Spasmodic dysmenorrhea is most frequent between the ages of 15 and 25 years. It ends abruptly after a full-term pregnancy, or it may end gradually with each period becoming less painful during the early twenties. The girl usually feels very well during the premenstruum, and then is suddenly doubled up with severe spasms of pain in the lower abdomen on the first day of menstruation. The pains are colicky in nature, coming about every 20 minutes and lasting about 5 minutes; in fact, they are similar to true labor pains. The girl obtains most relief curling up around a hot water bottle, and

Differences between Spasmodic and Congestive Dysmenorrhea

	Spasmodic	Congestive
Start of pain	First day of period	Up to 14 days before period
Site of pain	Lower abdomen, back, inner thighs	Lower abdomen, back, head, breasts, joints, and limbs
Type of pain	Comes in spasms	Heavy, dragging, and continuous, increasing as menstruation starts
Time of starting	2 years after menarche	Before menarche, after the pill, or at pregnancy
Usual age	15–25 years	13–53 years
Ovulation	Must be present	May be present or absent
Premenstrual symptoms	Absent	Present
Effect of stress	Unrelated	Increases symptoms
After pregnancy	Cured	Increased symptoms
Effect of pill	Cures	Increases symptoms
Treatment	Prostagladin inhibitors, estrogen, or the pill	Progesterone and a 3-hourly starchy diet

aspirin may help take the edge off the pain. The pain may become so severe that bed is the only refuge, and it may continue throughout the night, preventing sleep. A monthly absence from school or work is often necessary.

The pain is easier on the second day and is gone by the third or fourth day. The distribution of pain is in the "bikini" area, as shown in Figure 17; in fact it covers the area served by the uterine and ovarian nerves. The severity of the pain continues relentlessly on the first day of menstruation, month after month, and is not affected by stress. It may be helped, temporarily at least, by an operation popularly known as a "D & C," or dilatation and curettage, used to stretch the opening of the womb. The girl is often undeveloped, with sparse hair in her

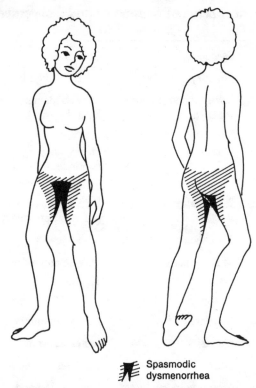

Spasmodic
dysmenorrhea

Figure 17 Site of pain in spasmodic dysmenorrhea

armpits and lower abdomen, small breasts with pink nipples, and acne.

It seems that spasmodic dysmenorrhea is caused by there being insufficient estrogen for maturing and stretching the muscles of the womb. During pregnancy there is an abundance of estrogen from the placenta for a full 9 months, and the muscle wall of the womb is stretched by the fetus. As a result, this type of period pain usually ends after pregnancy, and it is rare for the woman to subsequently suffer from premenstrual syndrome.

Sufferers of spasmodic dysmenorrhea are often advised to take more exercise or, alternatively, to relax more. As part of a survey for the British consumer magazine *Which?* some years ago, over 200 women with spasmodic dysmenorrhea kept a careful record of the pain they suffered for at least 3 cycles. As it happened, the survey took place in the summer when many were on vacation. The women who normally had active jobs, like waitresses or nurses, tended to choose restful vacations lying in the sun. The others who had more sedentary occupations chose active holidays, cycling 500 miles, mountaineering, and surfing. Regardless of their usual occupations or the amount of exercise they took, however, the amount of pain they experienced was not affected by the exercise or relaxation they had while on vacation.

When cells are damaged, a chemical called prostaglandin is released. In women with spasmodic dysmenorrhea, a high level of prostaglandin F-2-alpha is secreted by the cells of the lining of the womb. Certain drugs known as prostaglandin inhibitors are most effective in relieving this type of pain. (See page 195.)

CONGESTIVE DYSMENORRHEA

Congestive dysmenorrhea is the presence of heavy, continuous lower abdominal pain during the last 7 days of the premenstruum. The pain increases in severity on the first day of menstruation and then gradually eases, together with the end of the other premenstrual symptoms. The congestion was earlier thought to be due to water retention but is now recognized as a symptom of premenstrual syndrome. In contrast to spasmodic dysmenorrhea, sufferers of congestive dysmenorrhea may experience pain at their first menstruation and continue with it throughout their menstrual life, and the symptoms are present whether ovulation occurs or not. The pain is affected by stress, being worse when life in general is in a turmoil and being eased by happy events. A D & C brings no relief, nor does a pregnancy; in fact, because it is a premenstrual symptom it may become worse after each pregnancy. Again, in contrast to spasmodic dysmenorrhea, sufferers are more mature and physically developed, with large breasts and brown nipples. An interesting fact is that smoking tends to enhance the pain associated with symptoms in the premenstruum.

Estrogen administration increases the severity of premenstrual syndrome, which responds positively to progesterone. On the other hand, excess progesterone administered to girls who have not borne children can cause spasmodic dysmenorrhea. Thus, in theory, either type of dysmenorrhea can be produced at will by overdosing with the wrong hormone, estrogen or progesterone, which in itself proves that painful periods are not psychological but are caused by hormonal imbalance.

Despite the benefits that can be obtained by treating painful periods appropriately, certain women prefer not to ask for relief. I remember visiting a 19-year-old filing clerk who lived in a slum dwelling in a suburb in East London, for the flu. In conversation her mother mentioned that her daughter also suffered from severe period pains each month, and had to be brought home from the West End in a taxi. My immediate response was that suffering of this kind was no longer necessary and the pain could be treated, whereupon the girl replied, "Oh, don't! How else could I get a taxi ride once a month?"

MISPLACED CELLS

A rare cause of painful periods, which may occur with the first menstruation or after years of normal menstruation, and which affects about one woman in 20 who has dysmenorrhea, is due to a condition known as *endometriosis*. Cells of the lining of the cavity of the womb, or endometrium, become displaced, and may be found either in the muscle wall or outer coat of the womb itself; in the ligaments around the womb; in the ovary or tubes; in the bladder or bowel; or anywhere in the lower abdomen. (Figure 18 shows the relative position of the organs around the womb.) These cells lining the cavity of the womb have a unique ability to multiply, be shed, grow again, and multiply in an endless cycle under the influence of the menstrual hormones. Each time the lining cells are shed they pass out from the opening of the womb into the vagina and out of the body as a menstrual flow. However, the misplaced endometrial cells are not able to pass out of the body, and tend to accumulate as tiny cysts. In time these become inflamed, covered with scar tissue and adhesions. Each time thickening of the lining

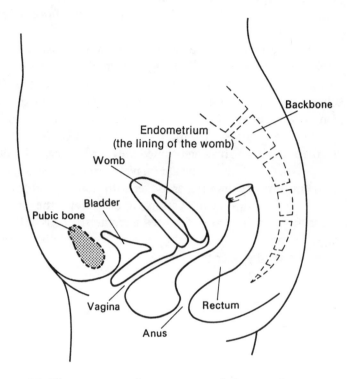

Figure 18 The position of organs around the womb

occurs during the premenstruum, these cysts become larger, and as the cells are shed at menstruation more room has to be found within these cysts for the extra cells. As you can imagine, after a time this creates a very painful condition. The pain is not limited to the bikini area but spreads all over the lower abdomen, possibly also affecting the bladder and rectum. In addition to causing painful periods, endometriosis is characterized by extreme pain during thrusting at intercourse, which may diminish all sexual desire, and also by infertility due to scar tissue forming around the ovaries and tubes. Doctors diagnose the condition by the patient's accounts of painful periods, pain at intercourse, infertility, and also by gynecological examination. If necessary they may do a laparascopy, an operation in which a minute periscope is inserted through a small cut in the abdominal wall, which allows the surgeon to see the tiny cysts and surrounding scar tissue.

Why the cells become displaced remains a mystery. It is possible that some were displaced during the developmental stage of the reproductive system in early fetal life. It is also possible that some lining cells find their way through the fallopian tubes into the pelvis, either at menstruation or during labor. The pain is absent during pregnancy, when there is no menstruation, although as mentioned previously, pregnancy does not often occur. The condition may be treated by stopping periods entirely for 9 months or longer with hormone treatment. This not only stops menstruation, it also stops the cyclical changes in the normal and displaced endometrial cells. Alternatively, the abnormal tissue and cysts may be surgically removed or burned away by laser treatment.

9

Awkward Adolescent

The menarche, or first menstruation, is an important milestone in any girl's life, and demonstrates that she has an intact hormonal pathway from the hypothalamus and pituitary to the ovaries and womb. It is heralded over a period of about two years by the appearance of secondary sex characteristics, such as breast development, skin and circulatory changes, the growth of pubic and armpit hair, and changes of the body shape into the rounded female figure. (See Figure 19.) It is not the end of pubertal development, however, and only represents about the halfway stage.

The changes in the breast occur very slowly, from the first development under the nipple of a small "bud" the size of a grape, through the gradual increase in size to full development. Often one breast develops slightly before the other, but although this inequality usually causes much worry and immediate medical advice is sought, there is no cause for alarm. In due course both breasts will develop equally, for the growth stimulus comes from hormones in the bloodstream.

In India and Sri Lanka the first menstruation is a cause for celebration, as it represents a girl's attainment of physical maturity and the beginning of her sexual and reproductive life. The occasion is marked by a change from wearing short dresses to dressing in colorful and beautiful saris. In Pakistan it is

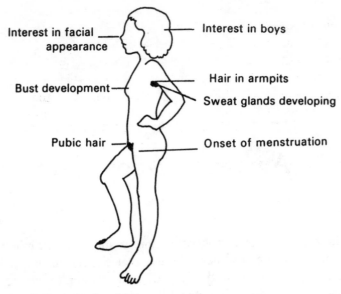

Figure 19 Female development at puberty

reported that the girls in some households are deliberately fed a low-protein diet in order to delay menarche, thus postponing the cost of the marriage that is expected to occur immediately after the menarche has taken place.

The attitude taken toward pubertal development depends very much on the culture and society to which a girl belongs. In societies such as Japan and Hong Kong, where the subject is still taboo, girls obtain information about their changes furtively, from the pages of popular magazines. In the U.S.A., on the other hand, sex education is discussed so freely at home, at school, and on the media, that when the menarche occurs it is almost a non-event. In any culture, however, the only girl in a male-dominated family may fear the menarche because it emphasizes the differences between her and her brothers, and may increase the conflict over her developing femininity.

The age of menarche is influenced by racial, genetic, dietetic, social, and economic factors. In Britain and the U.S.A. the average age of menarche is 13.1 years, but it varies throughout the world, being highest in the Bundi tribe in New Guinea at 18.8 years and lowest in Cuba at 12.4 years. Among British children attending special schools for the deaf and blind, menarche occurs early, at an average age of 12.2 years, and it is even earlier among those with congenital abnormalities that are known to start in early fetal life, like spina bifida and rubella, when the average is 10.8 years. On the other hand, the mentally disabled and those with Down's syndrome tend to have a later menarche. The usual age range for menarche is from 10 to 16 years—in fact, only 1 girl in a 100 has not started menstruating by the age of 16. There has been a trend for the age of menarche to decrease since 1850, when it was 17.5 years, and this decrease is attributed to better nutrition. It is thought that the age of menarche has stabilized in the last 25 years.

The first menstruation usually lasts between 3 and 8 days with an average of 5½ days, which is rather longer than most mothers expect it to be. Then there is usually an interval of 2 or 3 months before the next menstruation. Only about four menstruations occur during the first year after menarche, with the cycle gradually becoming shorter.

At 16 years of age, 20% of girls still have cycles that last longer than 40 days, and 33% have a prolonged bleeding lasting at least 7 days. Irregular menstruation is quite common for teenagers and there are many normal reasons for this, though it can be worrisome for the girl herself. In these years she is not only adjusting to her developing figure, she is also becoming more conscious of the opposite sex. As boyfriends come into the picture she becomes more interested in her own appearance and, all in all, these are often emotion-laden days.

In a single girl the cycle tends to be long, perhaps 35 days, but as she begins to be stimulated by contact with boyfriends her cycle may shorten by a few days and approach the conventional norm, for the menstrual hormones are stimulated by male contact. However, if the male contact is broken and she returns to female companionship, her cycle usually returns to its original pattern.

One 19-year-old inquired:

"My periods were always very irregular, with sometimes

even 8 weeks between them. When I first met John they became better, once as short as 28 days. Then we had an awful fight and I broke up with him. Since then, my cycles only seem to come when they want to, every 5 or 6 weeks. Does it matter?"

At 19 years old it does not matter, and probably even before she received a reply she would have found another boyfriend, and menstruation would have become more regular again.

Ovulation first occurs about 2 years after menarche, not necessarily every month initially, but every 2 or 3 months. Gradually, the cycles become more regular. It is with the onset of ovulation that spasmodic dysmenorrhea might begin. This usually comes as a surprise to both the girl and her mother, as previously menstruation had been so pain-free.

If the spasmodic dysmenorrhea is bad enough to need regular medication for the pain, especially if the girl has to take time off or stay in bed, then medical help should be sought. It is interesting to listen to mothers explain why they do not take their daughters to the doctor when the girls are suffering from spasmodic dysmenorrhea:

"I don't want to be considered fussy or neurotic."

"He'll only tell her to get married and have children like I was told!"

"I would hate her to have an operation."

"He might put her on the pill and she's too young for that—besides she hasn't any boyfriends yet."

"Boys would take advantage of her if she were on the pill."

Such attitudes are a great shame, because there is so much that can be done for these girls. If the parents do not want their daughter to have the pill, the doctor can always prescribe just estrogen, which is not a contraceptive by itself but will ease her monthly pains. Moreover, since the introduction of prostaglandin inhibitors, estrogen and the pill are no longer the only effective treatments available.

Even before the first menstruation, cyclical mood swings may occur and continue even at times of missed menstruation. (See Figure 6.) These mood swings can transform a happy schoolgirl into a lazy, bad-tempered, selfish grouch whose academic work and behavior deteriorate even before menstruation is established. As a pattern it is very suggestive of premenstrual syndrome, and the mood swings should be recorded so that help can be given to the girl before she falls too far behind in school.

These years may be marked by conflicts between the early maturers and those who mature more slowly. Long-term friendships may break up as one girl develops sooner than another. With maturation comes an interest in boys and a concern about appearance, so that endless time is spent in caring for the face and body. At this time, grease starts developing in the skin and the sweat glands begin to operate, so that skin care and deodorants become necessary.

Many girls do not like the body changes that Nature has decreed. They object to the rounded contours, and would prefer the broad shoulders and wiry limbs of boys. This stimulates the urge to diet, even in those who are not particularly overweight. Excessive dieting during these developing years is dangerous. It may halt menstruation and ovulation, and lead to *anorexia nervosa*, with weight-loss accompanied by food phobias and psychological changes. It is not unusual to find girls who reduce their weight from 120 pounds to 70 pounds within a few months by strict dieting, and still complain about their body and imagine that they are too fat. Unhappily, the road to recovery in such cases is slow and, if they develop multicystic ovaries, their future fertility is at stake. When menstruation does return, it is often accompanied by unpleasant premenstrual symptoms.

Unfortunately for many teenagers, these sexual developments may occur at just the same time as their mothers are experiencing the difficult years of menopause, and are also subject to mood swings and unpleasant symptoms. It is important to help adolescents through this stage, however, no matter how impossible and thoughtless they become. They need every opportunity to mix freely with older girls and women, and with boys and men, to help them sort themselves out and appreciate the differences in individual men and women.

Another concern is the increased sex desire that may occur premenstrually. This often causes problems for young adolescents, who are quite unprepared for this new sex urge and are unable to control their emotions. The increased sex drive may be responsible for young girls running away from home or custody, only to be found following boys in clubs and at school. These girls can be helped and their problem behavior frequently disappears if they receive appropriate treatment.

In puberty, premenstrual depression is usually worse than tiredness, and is likely to make a girl sulky, secretive, withdrawn, and anxious to be alone. Nevertheless, a careful watch should be kept on her behavior. Too often, the mood swings will occur suddenly, without warning or provocation, and she may make an unexpected suicide gesture.

> *Phyllis*, 17 years old, had been at the top of her class when she was 12, and her work had been the envy of others. Gradually, however, she went downhill in both work and behavior. She became sloppy, rude, and bored with everything, gave up any attempt at graduating from high school, and dropped out of school at the first opportunity. She first worked in a hairdressers' salon, but her work was unsatisfactory and her timekeeping poor. Her next job was as a filing clerk, where she felt unappreciated. There would be days when she would come home, slip up to her bedroom, and stay there for hours, allowing no one to enter and refusing food. One day her father found her in a corner apparently asleep. The doctor diagnosed an overdose of hypnotics and she had to be rushed to the hospital. This incident shocked her mother, who then started to keep a careful eye on her daughter. Soon she noted the correlation between her mood swings and menstruation, and asked for medical help. With treatment her daughter improved quickly, restarted her social life, which had been absent for 5 years, and later returned to night school.

Teenage girls with premenstrual syndrome should get proper

treatment, including progesterone if required. The need is usually only temporary; as they mature the need for regular medication decreases, although they may need it again in times of stress.

At one British boarding school, parents and visitors were invited to visit the dormitories on the annual Open Day. In each dormitory a grade sheet was displayed, showing the grade each girl had received for the tidiness of her bed and locker every morning. It was not difficult to determine the menstrual patterns of the girls by inspecting the grade sheets, for they were far more likely to receive a poor tidiness grade when they were exceptionally sleepy during the premenstruum.

At another boarding school, discipline books were used to record the names of girls and the date and reasons why they had been disciplined. These books were made available for analysis, together with the books the girls signed when they menstruated and needed sanitary protection. The study showed that during menstruation the girls had twice as many discipline problems as would normally be expected. Many of the incidents during menstruation could be accounted for by tiredness, and included offenses such as forgetfulness and unpunctuality. Other incidents reflected premenstrual irritability at having to conform to strict school discipline. Also, a girl is more likely to be punished for an offense during menstruation because she may be too slow to avoid detection. If several children are talking when the teacher enters the classroom, it will be those with a slow reaction time who will not stop talking quickly enough and will be caught.

This investigation also revealed two types of indiscipline. When it had been completed the principal, an exceptional woman who knew and was concerned with each individual girl, was shown two lists of girls' names and asked to comment on them. Unknown to her, the lists contained the names of the girls who had received the most punishments during the term. One list was those girls whose punishments had all occurred during the premenstruum. "Just naughty girls from exuberance or laziness; I'll probably be choosing a future class president from that list," she commented. But when shown the other list of girls whose punishments had occurred evenly throughout the menstrual cycle, she remarked, "They're the problem girls requiring careful handling and understanding," and she went on to describe how they had to cope with such difficulties as broken homes, immigrant parents, minor deformities, and so on.

In this study it was also noted that teachers' helpers, girls 16–18 years old who were permitted to discipline other girls for misbehavior, gave significantly more punishments during their own menstruations, and then their standard gradually relaxed through the rest of the cycle. This naturally raises a question about teachers, and indeed any women in positions of authority, such as judges and supervisors: do they give more punishments during their own menstruation? Are they more strict then? Or, once they become aware of the effect of menstrual hormones on their behavior, do they overcompensate to try to avoid being too severe when they themselves are menstruating?

As part of this survey, it was also possible to analyze how many days passed before a girl who had been punished once was punished a second time, a statistical method known as "critical event analysis." The results showed that most second punishments occurred within 4 days of the first offense, then there was a gradual decrease in further punishments until 25–28 days after the first offense, when there was an unexpected rise not only in those girls who were already menstruating, but also in girls who had not yet started menstruation. This suggests that these premenarche girls were already experiencing mood swings, a fact that many observant mothers had noticed in their daughters. A similar analysis was done in regard to boys at a nearby boarding school, but they did not show any evidence of cyclical mood swings at all.

On one occasion my adolescent daughter burst into the house from school asking for a menstrual chart. When asked why, she replied that her teacher had lost her temper and thrown a piece of chalk at a girl, and the same thing had occurred on the Thursday before semester break, exactly 4 weeks earlier!

When my daughter graduated from high school she passed on to the next class president a list of the probable dates of the teachers' menstruations, so that the students would know when to hand in their essays to get good grades.

In later years, when women meet and exchange memories, it is the unfair incidents and unjustified punishments that they remember best. One wonders how often these problems were caused by it being the wrong day of the month for the teachers.

School principals have a dual responsibility, to not only cope with their own premenstrual mood swings but also to recognize and deal with them in the girls whose education is entrusted to them. They should be ready to show understanding to girls who have episodes of irritability or become depressed, and give encouragement, particularly to prevent a girl from dropping out just because of some temporary difficulties.

As Figure 9 clearly shows, schoolgirls' work deteriorates during the premenstruum. A similar survey of women in the Armed Forces indicated lower intelligence scores in tests taken during the paramenstruum.

A study in 1968 on the effect of menstruation on the results of high school and college exams showed that those girls who were in their paramenstruum during exams had fewer passes, less honor grades, and a lower average grade. The girls whose results were most affected during the paramenstruum were those with cycles exceeding 31 days, and those whose menstruation lasted for 7 days or longer. In the high school exams some subjects were completed in 1 day, some had tests 4 days apart, and other subjects had tests at an interval of more than 8 days. The analysis showed that girls were at a greater disadvantage in those subjects where all tests were completed in 1 day (when they could be in their paramenstruum) in comparison with subjects where the exams were spaced more than 8 days apart, and they could not be entirely in their paramenstruum during both exams. It should be possible for examination boards and universities to arrange time-tables so that when two tests are necessary for a subject, they are 8 or more days apart.

At public examinations in England proctors may make a note at the top of the examination paper if a candidate is in her paramenstruum at the time of the exam. Of course, it is not known how much attention is paid to this fact by the examiners.

10

Marriage

The word "marriage" is used here in its broadest sense—the union of man and woman as true life partners—regardless of whether the union was solemnized in a religious ceremony, was legalized by being registered, or was a simple decision to live together. This chapter is not about social conventions; it is concerned with the impact of premenstrual syndrome on the lives of men, women, and children living together as families.

Perhaps the cynic who wrote: "Marriages are made in heaven, but they end up in hell!" was married to a woman who had a severe case of premenstrual syndrome. Or maybe he was just a keen observer of other people's marriages. Not all marriages end up in hell, of course, but for any young couple the stakes run pretty high, and if the woman suffers from premenstrual syndrome or develops it later, the problems will be more intense. Most men enter relationships utterly ignorant of the problems women face each month. The little knowledge they have is probably confined to a vague awareness of "periods," "bleeding," and "feminine hygiene products." If their mothers or their sisters suffered from PMS, they might have learned how to cope with it, but the odds are that they paid little attention and really know very little about the cause.

While they were going out together before the marriage, the girl may have avoided him on her difficult days. So, it is often not until they are living together that the problem emerges. If she suffers from spasmodic dysmenorrhea, he will probably be the first to see that she gets effective and complete relief from her pains, for pain is something he can understand. However, sudden mood swings, irrational behavior, and bursting into tears for no apparent reason may confuse him, and sudden aggression and violence, with no warning and little justification will shock and disturb him.

An article in the British magazine *Bride and Home* described what may lie ahead for the couple once the honeymoon is over:

> "Then quite suddenly you feel as if you can't cope anymore—everything seems too much trouble, the endless household chores, the everlasting planning of meals. For no apparent reason you rebel: 'Why should I do everything?' you ask yourself defiantly. 'I didn't have to do this before I was married. Why should I do it now?' Everything starts going wrong, and it gets worse instead of better.
>
> "As on other mornings, you get up and cook breakfast while your husband is in the bathroom. You climb wearily out of bed and trudge down the stairs, a vague feeling of resentment growing within you. The sound of cheerful whistling from upstairs only makes you feel a little more cross. Without any warning the toast starts to scorch, and the sausages, instead of happily sizzling in the pan, start spitting and spluttering furiously. Aghast, you rescue the toast, which by this time is beyond resurrection and fit only for the trash. The sausages are charred relics of their former selves and you throw those out too. Your unsuspecting husband opens the kitchen door expecting to find his breakfast ready and waiting, only to see a smoky atmosphere and a thoroughly overwrought wife. You are so dismayed at him finding you in such chaos that you just burst helplessly into tears."

What is the young husband going to make of this situation? Much depends upon his family background. If he encountered similar situations at home before marriage, he will probably react as he did then. If he is used to making himself scarce and getting out of the house, he'll probably grab his things and dash for the office, leaving his wife to sort out her troubles. If he was in the habit of helping to sort out the chaos, he'll probably sympathize with her, give her a kiss, make her a cup of coffee and breakfast, and insist on her going back to bed for the day. Obviously, this is the wisest course of action.

But what if he has never encountered this sort of thing before? How will he cope? Will he ignore it, hoping that it is only a temporary lapse until, once a month, month after month, it recurs? Or will he rage about breakfast being ruined and storm out of the house, to arrive at work hungry and unable to do his work properly, eventually returning home tired and frustrated to an equally distraught wife? Not a happy omen.

Fortunately, not all women suffer from PMS, and not all PMS sufferers become hellcats. Someone should educate the husband-to-be about the problems that can arise, how to recognize them, and what treatments are available to provide complete relief.

So far in this chapter we have been considering the situation of a newlywed woman with premenstrual syndrome. Often, however, premenstrual syndrome does not start until after a pregnancy. Just imagine the situation. The couple have enjoyed their life together for a year or more, until the baby came along, and now once a month there are the frustrations, mood swings, irritability, and apparent laziness—in addition to having to cope with the baby. Once, he could do nothing wrong; now he finds he can do nothing right on those terrible days. If he has been observant, and kept track of her menstrual dates, he may soon recognize the time relationship. Realizing the importance of food, especially frequent starchy snacks for those with premenstrual syndrome, he should keep a careful eye on her eating habits. On the other hand, if neither of them has any clear idea of her menstrual dates, they will probably go on fighting month after month until they can't stand it any longer.

All this suffering is quite unnecessary, and a tragic destruction of family life. The answer lies in the true nature of marriage, which is that both partners share equally in every aspect of their lives. If, when their relationship becomes serious, they both discuss the issue, and keep a chart of her menstruation and any symptoms that she has, they will soon realize when things are going wrong. That is the time to seek medical advice and obtain treatment. Keeping the chart together will help them to understand each other better, and the man will have a much greater understanding of what menstruation means to a woman. He may also find that he is the first to notice the warning signs of premenstrual syndrome, such as a slight irrationality of conversation, or lack of conversation, and the minor disagreements in which there is a certain rigidity in her views. More important still is the darkening of the skin around the eyes, one of the surest signs that she is about to enter her premenstruum. In some women the skin goes so dark as to appear almost black.

If they have children, he should remember that they are more likely to get out of hand when their mother is less able to care for and play with them. He should try to be a substitute mother as well as a father, as best as he can. He should remember that there is housework to be done, and it is no use telling her to rest—if the work has to be done and there is no one else to do it, she will not rest. A neighbor or a relative could be asked to help; it will probably only be for 4 or 5 days, unless the symptoms are very severe. Once menstruation has started, and while events are still fresh in their minds, they should discuss whether she is getting adequate medical help, and he should assure her that he will support her. More husbands accompany their wives to the doctor or hospital when asking for help for premenstrual syndrome than for any other gynecological condition, including infertility.

The following excerpts from letters reveal how often the husband is involved with his wife's premenstrual syndrome:

> "I am fortunate in having a very understanding husband who puts up with my tirades as best he can, but he says he sometimes doesn't know how to cope with me."

> "My husband first noticed the connection with my menstrual cycle without mentioning it to me 18 months ago, and backs me up completely in writing to you."

"The misery has gone on for years, misery and misery. Seventeen jobs in ten years. Now I clean offices, and for two weeks out of the month my husband gets up at 4 A.M. and does them for me."

Frequently, husbands devise their own means of confirming the diagnosis beforehand; thus the computer manager came to the clinic complete with a computer print-out to prove it, while a draftsman turned up with a beautifully drawn blueprint; others merely bring along the office diary or kitchen calendar.

There are still too many husbands out there who have not made the diagnosis, or who do not realize that help is available. They may know when they wake up that it's going to be one of those days, and no matter what they do, they will not be able to satisfy her. If he returns home with red roses she'll ask, "Why didn't you bring me my favorite chocolates?" but when he brings the right kind of chocolates it'll be, "You know I'm dieting, how can you be so cruel?" He just can't win.

The monthly problems can interfere with their social life and even with his earning capacity. Some years ago, a door-to-door salesman was sent by his employer for medical help. He worked on commission, and while his average weekly commission was quite high, one week in four his earnings fell drastically. Not only did he find it difficult to plan his spending, but his chances of promotion were being affected. He explained to the doctor that he became more depressed and seemed to start work later during the weeks when his earnings were low, and he could not explain why. When asked about his wife's menstruation, however, the connection dawned on him. A few days later he brought along his wife's menstrual record, which confirmed that premenstrual irritability and tiredness were affecting him. She was delighted to be offered progesterone treatment, and responded well. Her husband was also delighted when he got a promotion.

Marital conflict is a recurring theme among those seeking medical help:

"My marriage broke up 7 years ago, and I feel this trouble was a big cause of the break-up. I have since turned down a chance to remarry, as I cannot face burdening someone else with my continual monthly problems."

"This premenstrual misery is a very real threat to the survival of our marriage."

"We have been married for 8 years, during which time my premenstrual tension has been a constant problem. During the past 3 years this has become more acute and increasingly more severe, with a traumatic effect on our relationship and on our two boys of 5 and 3 years."

"My husband has urged me to write; our marriage is breaking up, my children are suffering, and after 5 years of my trouble my poor husband can take no more."

"My husband has already left me, and I have two children with whom I try hard not to lose my temper at this time, but I feel sorry for them; it is really awful."

"I have come to dread my periods, and even my husband rushes to the calendar at an unexpected outburst on my part. I get violent with my husband."

Sometimes the marital disharmony just manifests as silence, on other occasions there are vicious verbal battles, and, at the extreme limit, fights and batterings. How may wives batter their husbands during their paramenstruum is unknown, nor do we know how often the husband is provoked by her premenstrual anger and batters her.

One mother wrote about a daughter who was receiving treatment for premenstrual irritability and food cravings:

"Some cakes and cookies I had been saving for a party disappeared on Sunday. It was all too much for me and I burst into tears. This in turn upset my husband, who went and found Mary in her bedroom and gave her a thrashing. At midnight we discovered she was missing. She had spent the night with friends. Both Mary and I started menstruating that day."

This is also a case of menstrual synchrony, where the mother's and daughter's menstruation occur at the same time, and where the mother's distress caused the husband to take it out on his daughter.

Two researchers in Washington, D.C., Roger Langley and Richard Levy, have estimated that there are 12 million battered husbands in the United States. They believe it is the "most unreported crime," affecting 20% of husbands. Again, one wonders how often the wives were also victims of their own hormonal imbalance.

A couple of letters suggest that the premenstruum may frequently be the cause:

> "I attacked him with a carving knife on one occasion, and another time while building a stone wall I lifted huge stones and threw them at him."

> "I have tried to knife my husband too many times to count ... but for one fantastic week I feel on top of the world."

Most marriage guidance counselors are well aware of the traumas that can be caused to the marital relationship by premenstrual syndrome, and try to let the partner know about this. Often, when telephoned urgently for help because of a big fight, a wise counselor will arrange a meeting 7 days later, when the woman is more likely to be in her postmenstrual phase, will have more insight and will be more open to reason.

For most of the month, a housewife works all day in the home, dealing with the cooking, cleaning, shopping, laundry, ironing, and perhaps even the gardening. On certain days, though, it may all become too much. She may feel too apathetic to cope with the chores, avoids the cooking, and leaves the house untidy. Alternatively, she may have a spurt of restless energy, and obsessively clean and polish everything until she wears herself out. Then she may blame her premenstrual symptoms on the fact that she "overdid it." One difficulty facing the woman who is at home all day is the temptation to miss meals, waiting to enjoy a meal with her husband at night. The busier she is, the quicker time passes, and the longer the intervals between food. During the paramenstruum this can result in the problems caused by low blood sugar levels.

The woman who also works away from the home faces different problems. In an effort to control herself in front of her fellow workers, and possibly also the public, she may hold back her frustrations until she reaches home—then lets go at her nearest and dearest. Again, she may well have missed her lunch and gone a long interval without food, not appreciating the problems this causes.

An important problem the couple must face is that of sexual harmony. Dr. Ruth D'arcy Hart, Medical Officer at the Fertility and Problems Clinic in London, found that 60% of married women noted that their sex urge was greatest before menstruation. Unfortunately for those with premenstrual syndrome, this is also the time at which many of them are least approachable, feel most unloved, and out of anger, may refuse their husbands' sexual overtures. (Incidentally, one of the side effects of the pill that is too rarely mentioned is its ability to decrease the natural sex urge.) Satisfactory sex between partners is the best cement for any marriage. There is much that can be done these days if difficulties develop in this area, and it is really worthwhile seeking help. One cause of a decrease in sexual satisfaction which has only recently been recognized, but is most responsive to treatment, is the loss of sex urge that occurs after a pregnancy complicated by postnatal depression. A blood test may show the wife to have a raised prolactin level, in which case treatment with bromocriptine can help.

Men do not have cycles akin to women. On page 88 a "critical event analysis" is described which detected cycles of indiscipline in premenarcheal girls. Similar analyses have been done on surveys of disciplinary incidents among prisoners and schoolboys, and on symptoms of glaucoma in men and women. The results were similar, except that in the women there was a return of the critical event after an interval of 25–28 days whereas the men showed no such return, suggesting that if men do have a cycle it is quite different from a woman's.

Margaret Henderson of Australia has shown that some men have an ovulation temperature chart that is synchronous with their wives' charts. When the wife has a mid-cycle temperature drop followed by a rise at ovulation lasting for 12–14 days until she menstruates, the husband also has a temperature drop followed by a rise, although the temperature does not stay up. However, if the wife has an anovular cycle, with no drop and rise at ovulation, the husband's chart follows hers and he does not show an ovular rise. If the wife goes on the pill or becomes pregnant, and so stops ovulating, again the husband does not have the characteristic drop and rise. If the man moves out to live alone, or with another man, again the characteristic drop and rise will be lost. Although this work remains unproven it does suggest that close companionship and harmony between a couple can lead to their bodies' rhythms becoming synchronous, with the man following the woman's cycle pattern.

As mentioned earlier, many husbands accompany their wives to the doctor's office if she is suffering from premenstrual syndrome, and others usually agree to come to the next interview. This is a most valuable opportunity for them to learn more about the full extent of their wives' problems. At the same time much useful information can be given to them to help them to cope better. First, a husband must understand what premenstrual syndrome is, why it occurs, and the importance of a dietary regimen. Second, he should appreciate which of his wife's symptoms *can* be helped, and which ones are not premenstrual but occur throughout the month and therefore are not likely to benefit from progesterone treatment. He should be taught how to chart the symptoms, and may want to keep his own chart of events. Often, the husband is the first to realize that his wife could use some extra progesterone, and it may be possible to give the couple permission to raise the dose when they jointly feel it is needed. The husband should also understand the problems brought on by low blood sugar levels; that his wife will feel worse if she is deprived of sleep; and that during the premenstruum, her desire for alcohol may increase but she will become intoxicated on half her usual amount. If she already has a tendency toward excessive consumption of alcohol then this is a time for him to give special care and support.

If the husband really understands the situation, he will be much more able to help make the necessary adjustments to their life. Quite a few men phone home at regular intervals to ensure that their wives are eating regularly. One, realizing his wife's irritability in the premenstruum, asked the bank manager to send their joint balance sheets on specified days, so that they could discuss financial arrangements calmly in her postmenstruum. During the premenstruum, when the wife has little insight, decisions about stressful things such as moving, holidays, and schools should be delayed by a week or so. If help is needed in the home it may be better to arrange this for the one special week of the month rather than the usual one day per week.

How much responsibility should a husband have for his wife's premenstrual violence? In addition to ensuring that his wife receives medical treatment, and providing for the care of the children and the home when she is most vulnerable, does he have a responsibility for the protection of the public? Should he report her violence to some appropriate authority? In fact, who _is_ the appropriate authority? What are his responsibilities if her violence brings her into conflict with the law? Too often such cases are reported too late, when the woman is already charged with the assault, baby battering, or murder, and the husband in her defense produces disturbing stories of her cyclical problems. All these questions need serious consideration, for at present there are no clear guidelines to help the unfortunate family in such desperate circumstances.

It is regrettable that successive cultures over the centuries have encouraged the idea that women are enigmas, with problems they can only resolve themselves, and that they should just get on with it. Today we recognize that such ideas are apocryphal legacies of the past, but attitudes change slowly, and only when men have a more complete understanding of women's problems will any real progress be made.

11

❧

Advice For Men

Premenstrual syndrome is a man's problem too. With about 40% of women suffering from premenstrual syndrome, the law of averages ensures that sooner or later a man will find himself on the receiving end. It could be his mother, sister, partner, girl-friend, any woman in his workplace or anywhere else. If he has not learned to handle the situation and doesn't know where to get help, then it could be a very traumatic experience indeed.

It is often said that if men suffered from premenstrual syndrome they would soon find a cure. Well, men do suffer from the effects of premenstrual syndrome on the women with whom they come into contact, either at work or at play. It has been so for thousands of years, yet they are mighty slow at recognizing it, diagnosing it, and understanding the treatment required. Usually, those men who do suffer do not discuss it with other men, and therefore feel they are dealing with an exceptional, unpredictable, or difficult woman. When they do talk to other men they are surprised to find that many have similar problems, and some are even worse off.

MALE REACTION

Only those who have encountered the suddenly changed personality of a woman severely affected by premenstrual syndrome and have come face to face with her unreasonableness and anger can have any idea of the trauma and the sense of unreality about what is happening that this brings. As the emotion of this irrational situation sweeps away common sense and reason, feelings of numbness and impotence take over. The man's thinking becomes disjointed and incoherent, he feels powerless and immobilized by the flood of abuse that submerges his own personality, until in sheer confusion and desperation he runs away.

This situation is graphically presented in the Introduction to this book, in the excerpt from David Duff's book _Albert & Victoria_. It vividly portrays the reactions of Queen Victoria's husband and ministers, showing their confusion and inability to cope when faced with an irrational premenstrual outburst from a woman who was their queen, but whose tension, irritability, changing moods, violence, and periods of negative attitudes were quite incomprehensible to them. They were all baffled, unsure of what they should do, and quite unable to deal effectively with the situation.

The reaction of Albert, the Prince Consort, was to try logical arguments. Like many other men, he did not appreciate or understand the unreasoned emotion that surged like a maelstrom in Queen Victoria's brain. He did not realize that one cannot talk logic to an illogical mind, and that that is the state of the premenstrual syndrome sufferer at such a moment.

Even Lord Melbourne, "a past master at dealing with women," was unable to handle the situation, to say nothing of the poor cabinet minister who simply fled, too frightened to even follow the correct protocol for leaving the queen's presence. Here were three men, presumably of high intelligence, so greatly affected by their situation yet unable to take any positive action or do anything to prevent a recurrence. Who knows how many other people in the course of history have faced similar situations and not had the knowledge to do anything about them.

Ten years earlier, Charles Lamb, the great English essayist, had died. For some 25 years he had been at the receiving end of recurrent attacks of premenstrual violence by his sister, Mary Lamb, during one of which she killed their mother. With great loyalty and courage Charles Lamb took upon himself the burden of responsibility for his sister's care. With her consent, he would lock her up in a special closet each month at the time of her attacks. He was rewarded with her lifelong affectionate devotion, for she kept house for him and helped with his writings, which also shows her postmenstrual normalcy.

Similar events occur daily all around us, yet most of us turn a blind eye to them. Is it not time that men decided to learn more about this disease and the way to handle it? It has been suggested that this is a disease of twentieth-century civilization, but this is only true to the extent that the media today exploit it, and it offers a chance for profit to quacks and entrepreneurs.

Premenstrual syndrome has been around for thousands of years. As mentioned before, Hippocrates in 400 B.C. suggested that it was caused by "agitated blood trying to find a way out of the body." A century earlier Simonides of Ceos, the Greek poet, wrote a classic poem about the changing moods of women, which he likened to the changing moods of the sea. This image provides an unmistakable representation of the sudden personality changes of the premenstrual woman.

MEN ARE DIFFERENT

"Why can't a woman be more like a man?" explodes Professor Higgins in My Fair Lady, Lerner & Lowe's adaptation of George Bernard Shaw's Pygmalion. Thousands of men must have felt like this when faced with their fair lady's attacks of premenstrual syndrome. Professor Higgins' outburst can be taken in two ways: either as a frustrated protest, or as a serious question. Nature, having planned males and females for different functions in reproduction, has also ensured that a woman cannot behave like a man, and vice versa. Men and women are different but equal. What is more, it is impossible for a man to experience what a woman has to go through as a consequence of her role in Nature's plan. There is no way that a healthy man can have any idea of what it is like to be unable to control his actions or behavior at certain times of the month, as is the case for a few women with premenstrual syndrome. So what can he do to help? He needs to be aware of her problems, and to be sympathetic and supportive during the premenstrual days. He should realize and reassure her that help is available and that there is no reason for her to suffer unnecessarily. Now that the hormonal background of premenstrual syndrome is becoming increasingly understood, there is so much more that can be done to control and eliminate the suffering.

RECOGNIZE THE EARLY SIGNS

Some men remain unaware of the problem until they awaken one morning to a hysterical and completely irrational woman with whom it is impossible to reason, and who may become violent. This is recognizing premenstrual syndrome the hard way. Others, who are more observant, may gradually become aware of her changing moods. She may become pessimistic, negative, and withdrawn at times, and nothing can be done to please her. She may be snappy, argumentative, impatient, and illogical; or she may shout, shriek, yell, and swear. She may even be violent, ready to bang on the table, slam doors, throw plates, vases, and books, kick the dog or cat, or hit those nearest and dearest to her, which means you and your children.

This emphasizes the need of keeping a menstrual chart (see page 24) to keep track of these mood changes. Frequently, it is the man in her life who first makes the connection and recognizes a woman's menstrual cyclicity. Not every sufferer from PMS knows she has the disease. She may believe her mood swings are caused by an explosive personality, and are something that cannot be changed, in which case a menstrual chart will help her to realize where the symptoms come from.

During her premenstruum, a woman may change her likes and dislikes of food, clothes, or furnishings. You may return from work to find the room changed around, or in the process of being rearranged and left for you to finish. She may have food binges, alcoholic urges, and spending sprees, buying things she does not need, clothes that do not fit, and food she never eats.

Some women have "lazy" days when they would rather not exert themselves. Others have "energetic" days when they will not sit down and are forever tidying up and finding more jobs to do. Yet others have "urgent" days when everything must be done today, immediately, not tomorrow or next week. No two women are alike.

A few women become paranoid during the premenstruum, and accuse their partner of all sorts of outrageous behavior, often suspecting an affair. These are the "unforgetting and unforgiving" days, but they, too, will pass. Some have "jealousy" days, which recur monotonously each cycle. Until she is treated it is best to accept this. Don't protest, but try not to show any interest in other women. It is also no use arguing logically during the premenstruum; just wait until the postmenstruum when she will be calmer and ready to listen—although she may then be tormented with guilt at her earlier behavior.

Perhaps the most difficult thing to understand is that just when women are most unbearable is often also the time when some of them most enjoy sex. It may sound contradictory and incomprehensible, but that just gives some idea of the irrationality that accompanies the hormonal upset.

How to Cope

The most important piece of advice during her difficult time: don't reason, discuss, or argue with her. Above all, keep control of yourself, and try not to become angry. Remember that premenstrual syndrome is an illness, a disease. Don't say, "Of course! It's the wrong time of the month!" Don't show her the menstrual chart, which will prove you are right. *Do* keep reassuring her of your concern, support, and love; she needs this, even though she may reject it. Try especially to help her to eat a little, and often. Find her favorite snacks and make sure there are plenty around. Don't worry if she has an eating binge: it is a sign that the sugar stores in her body are seriously depleted and she needs to replenish them. Instead, try to make sure it is her last binge by getting her to eat some starchy food every 3 hours. (See Chapter 16.) Discourage her from starting on a weight-loss diet until her premenstrual syndrome has been properly treated. Admire her good qualities, but don't mention her weight, or tease her about her figure. If necessary, phone her during the day to ensure that she is eating something regularly, or ask a neighbor to check on her. If she likes alcohol, she may experience very strong urges to drink during this time, so keep an eye on the home supplies and if they are disappearing too rapidly then remove all alcohol from the home.

Explain to your children that Mother is not well today. If possible, arrange for a neighbor, friend, or member of the family to take care of them for a day or even for a few hours. The opportunity will always arise for you to repay the kindness. Children can also be very helpful in ensuring that Mother eats regularly if you give them the necessary instructions and leave the food in a convenient place.

Use these difficult days to learn all you can about premenstrual syndrome. Make an appointment to see the doctor with her when she is in the postmenstruum. Doctors are often more sympathetic about premenstrual syndrome when the partner accompanies the patient. Remember to take the menstrual chart with you; it is the only thing the doctor needs to make a firm diagnosis. Tell the doctor how it is affecting your life as well as hers. Find out about local support or self-help groups. Many support groups encourage partners, and if your group does, then take advantage of it. You may be surprised to find that other men suffer even more than you.

When peace and tranquillity return in the postmenstruum, show her the menstrual chart you have been keeping, and discuss its implications. Explain that you understand what is happening, encourage her to see her doctor, and, most importantly, remind her that there is satisfactory treatment available. If possible, discuss the importance of the 3-hourly starchy diet and start with it right away. Remember that it must be rigidly adhered to every day of the month.

If it is necessary for her to have progesterone treatment, learn all about it, and see that she takes it as instructed. If she is allowed to increase the dose when needed, then you will probably be the first to realize when that time comes. If she is a candidate for progesterone injections, consider if you can give them. It is not difficult to do.

When men learn to recognize premenstrual syndrome and understand how to help sufferers, then there will be no need for them to be on the receiving end. Harmony will return to the household, and women will be happier and better able to cope with their life.

12

❧

Mother

The mother is the linchpin of the family. When her life is made miserable each month by the effects of premenstrual syndrome, it affects the whole family: husband, babies, schoolchildren, and teenagers. Children, even infants of only a few months, are very sensitive to changes in their mother's mood. If they cannot understand the reason for a change, they will react to it in their own peculiar way.

When you ask adult sufferers of premenstrual syndrome if their mother also suffered in the same way, you are likely to get many positive—and some rather interesting—replies, such as:

"We used to say, 'The dragon's on the warpath,' and we all knew what it meant. But it only lasted a day or two."

"I remember my brother putting up a red flag on the front door to warn us to be careful in our approach to mother."

Health professionals and social workers soon recognize when one of the mothers in their care is in her premenstruum. The usually tidy house is not picked up, the beds aren't made, dirty dishes sit on the kitchen table, and there is probably a burned cake by the sink. Perhaps the children went off to school late, in yesterday's clothes, and chances are that the meals will not be ready on time.

Although PMS may start at puberty, it can also begin—or get worse—after the children are born, especially if there is any depression after childbirth. This was a recurring theme in many letters:

> "Since the birth of my last child 2 years ago (I have five children), I have changed from being a normal housewife and mother to an unpredictable, bad-tempered person. During my period, my moods make me feel positively ill, especially my head. If only I could grow a new one, I say to my husband."

> "I have had attacks of depression since the birth of my first child, and I have never regained confidence in myself since then."

> "After the baby's birth I changed, and now I get an incredible amount of head pressure for a few days prior to the bleeding. It feels as though the top of my head is about to blow off with pressure. I spoke to my doctor about the possibility of an early menopause starting, but he only smiled and said it was more likely premenstrual tension."

> "I have a 22-month-old son, and I cannot remember feeling like this before he was born. I love him very much, but the poor little soul does have a terrible time when I shout at him and make him sob his heart out. I seem unable to stop, although I feel terrible about what I'm doing. It's almost as though I must be getting some sort of pleasure from it, and I feel very, very upset and guilty afterwards."

Dr. Christine Cooper, a pediatrician, has stated that children can be psychologically damaged for life by verbal violence.

The sudden onset of irritability after the birth of a child may surprise many mothers, who did not experience it before. They find themselves becoming quick-tempered and making totally irrational decisions. They become impatient with the children, not waiting for them to learn to dress or eat for themselves. They become intolerant, won't accept that "kids will be kids," shout at them when they are playing harmlessly, and complain that the children won't behave. They are like the school-teacher's helpers who expected a higher standard of discipline when they themselves were menstruating.

When a mother has a great deal to do it's easy for her to miss her own meals while feeding the family; alternatively she may be dieting. Unfortunately, her irritable and aggressive outbursts are likely to occur when her blood sugar level is at its lowest, which makes matters even worse. (See pages 149–152.)

> _Rose,_ an intelligent, unmarried 24-year-old mother, contacted the National Society for the Prevention of Cruelty to Children, as she feared she might harm her 6-year-old son during her premenstruum. It was obvious from her story that she had come very close to hurting him. She described her usual day: "Getting up at 8:00 A.M. and having a meal of toast and coffee together, then walking half a mile to his school, doing the shopping on the way home, then housework until it was time to pick him up from school at 3:30 P.M." This was the worst time of the day, and just before her periods she would feel aggressive as she met him. Suddenly a surge of hatred would well up and if he didn't behave, this is when he would be beaten.

In fact, Rose was describing how she became angry toward her son 7½ hours after her last meal, having used a lot of energy during the interval. Her menstrual chart confirmed that she lost her temper only during the premenstruum. Since she has started receiving treatment with progesterone and eating a midday meal and regular snacks every day, she has been happier and trouble-free. Rose also began to mark in advance on her menstrual chart the days on which she had to exert extra self-control, because she was anxious to do the best she could for her son.

Two remarks I often hear after successful treatment of a patient are, "Even my children behave better," and, "They don't shout so much nowadays." Some doctors even write in their files "CBB" meaning "children behaving better." In fact, children respond quicker to their mother's improved temper than do cats or dogs, who take a long time to forget ill-treatment.

Contraception often proves a problem for those with premenstrual syndrome, because they are liable to have side effects on the pill. Unfortunately, tubal ligation, previously thought to be a convenient permanent solution, has been shown to reduce the blood progesterone level. If they are receiving progesterone, this can be used contraceptively, as discussed on pages 210–211.

CHILDREN CANNOT UNDERSTAND

Children, who cannot understand their mother's mood swings, may react by developing psychosomatic or bodily symptoms such as a cough, runny nose, endless crying, temper tantrums, or vomiting. In my general practice when children were brought in with such complaints, the mother was given one chart on which to record the dates of the child's symptoms and another on which to record the dates of her own menstruation. When she returned with the charts after 2 or 3 months, it was surprising how often they clearly showed that the child was reacting with various ailments to the mother's mood swings. A survey of 100 mothers visiting the doctor because their child had a cough or cold showed that 54% of the mothers were in their paramenstruum. The children who were brought during the mother's paramenstruum tended to be under 2 years, only children, those with symptoms of less than 24 hours' duration, and those whose mothers were under 30 years of age. One girl was only 9 months, yet her mother brought a chart showing that for each time she had menstruated in the previous 3 months the child had developed a cough and runny nose.

A 6-month-old girl with herpes (or shingles) on her knee was brought to the office by her mother, who had had recurrent premenstrual herpes on her upper lip for several years.

Another survey was carried out among children who were admitted as emergencies to the North Middlesex Hospital in London. The mothers of 100 children were interviewed, and the results were very similar: in fact, 49% of the mothers were in their paramenstruum on the day the child was admitted. Some were admitted because of illness such as asthma, abdominal pain, or a temperature of unknown cause, while others had been injured in an accident. If the mother is accident-prone during her paramenstruum, the children in her care are also accident-prone. And if she is tired during the paramenstruum, she may not notice little Johnny running toward an oncoming car or climbing a dangerous tree, and so he will be in even greater danger then.

One day a telephone call informed me that an 18-month-old boy had had a high temperature and a convulsion. This was the third convulsion at intervals of 3–4 weeks. Inquiry revealed that it was not related to the mother's menstrual cycle but to his Nanny, who had total care of the boy while his mother worked full time. There had been some trouble with the Nanny the day before, and she had just given notice. The two previous convulsions had occurred at the time of Nanny's paramenstruum.

SIBLING JEALOUSY

Sometimes a situation is incorrectly diagnosed as jealousy of a brother or sister, when the real diagnosis is premenstrual syndrome in the mother.

Susan, 30 years old, had felt very well during her second pregnancy, with plenty of energy so that she would take 3-year-old David out each afternoon to play on the swings or kick a ball around in the nearby park. She had an easy delivery of a much-wanted daughter, but afterward became so depressed that she needed psychiatric treatment. David had been dry since the age of 16 months, but after his sister's birth he gradually started to wet the bed again, not every night, but in batches every few weeks. It seemed easy to blame it on jealousy of the new baby, but when Susan kept a careful record it showed that David's bedwetting was occurring during her premenstruum. Susan admitted that she "hadn't been the same" since the baby's birth, and had been too tired and busy to take David for his usual play-time in the park.

BATTERED CHILDREN

The most tragic aspect of premenstrual syndrome is when it becomes so severe that the mother, in a state of confusion and rage, batters her beloved child. These mothers, contrary to popular belief, are women who often really love their children. They have strong maternal feelings, but in a sudden moment of premenstrual irritability they lose control and harm their offspring.

A social worker's report on a 35-year-old mother of two children reads:

> "During the last premenstruum her youngest daughter, aged 18 months, was screaming and would not stop. Patient was very irritated by this and picked her up and squeezed her—this started a circle of louder screaming and harder squeezing until patient 'heard something crack.' She was immediately frightened and threw the child on the floor and sat crying on the chair. When more composed, she examined Joan and took her to the doctor."

This type of injury to a child is, tragically, not uncommon. Judging from the letters and stories of my patients, the cases of baby-battering that are reported are only the tip of the iceberg.

> "Because I lost my temper and hit my eldest child when he was 4, just before a period, I nearly had a complete nervous breakdown. Even though I feel much better now, my premenstrual tension remains, and from day 18 of the cycle until day 4 of my period I suffer from depression, temper, forgetfulness, and dizziness."

> "It has gotten to a stage now that every month something the children do triggers me off. It is as though there is somebody inside me saying terrible things. I blame my son and tell him I hate him, and hit him. Sometimes he gets out of my way quickly."

If the situation becomes worse, the children may be taken into care, but this is a drastic step. One wonders about the aftereffects on the many slightly battered children, who are not referred to social services and are not helped. Does the unsettled, temperamental background of such a childhood leave any scars, such as shyness or lack of confidence?

A woman who had been treated with progesterone for 17 years was asked if she would like to take part in a television program dealing with PMS. She went home and explained to her family that she couldn't recall those far-off days. "You must be joking! Dad and I will never be able to forget your vicious temper," was the comment from her daughter, now in her twenties.

A 35-year-old teacher married to the principal of a school stated:

> "For 7 days during the premenstruum I become tense, irritable, shouting, weepy and tired, bloated with swelling of my legs and ankles, and with headaches over my eyes. I have two children and at those times when I am in an uncontrollable temper, I have hit them really hard."

She was successfully treated with progesterone for 12 months and has been free from symptoms since. She later wrote:

> "It has been a valuable experience—I would never have believed that an intelligent woman like me, with high morals and a good education, could ever lose control of herself to such an extent that she would batter her children, for I love my children dearly. How utterly illogical it is that I personally should cause them permanent harm."

When the child reaches school, the teacher may notice that absences seem to occur at regular intervals. One 10-year-old girl was referred for treatment by her teacher, who noticed absences for a few days at the beginning of each month. The teacher wondered if it was because of the girl's menstruation, but, in fact, it was because her mother had recurrent premenstrual asthma requiring rest in bed, and the daughter was kept at home to answer the door.

TEENAGERS' REACTIONS

Truancy from school may also be related to a mother's premenstrual symptoms, as in the case of one mother who wrote:

> "For days before a period starts I hate everyone and make the family's life a misery. My 13-year-old daughter will not go to school when I'm like this. She is frightened of what I may do, and cries when I start drinking."

Teenagers, both boys and girls, are quick enough to spot the changes in their mother and notice when she's "in one of those moods." As one boy put it, "Our whole life revolves around Mom's periods."

The mother's problem is not helped when the daughter starts to menstruate, especially if both periods occur together in synchrony. Many mothers, recognizing the problem in themselves, seek help for their daughter's premenstrual syndrome. They may feel that they've weathered the storm so far, and it won't be long before the end, but they are not prepared to let their daughters suffer as they have done.

Finally, all mothers, and fathers too, have the responsibility of seeing that their children receive a good sex education, especially about those problems that come back once a month.

13

The World's Workers

The cost to industry because of menstrual problems is high and is measured in millions of pounds, liras, kroners, and dollars, as well as in terms of human misery, unhappiness, and pain. It has been estimated to cost U.S. industry 8% of its total wage bill, compared with 5% in Sweden, 3% in Italy, and 3% in Britain. The load is not spread evenly, for the industries that suffer most are those employing large numbers of women, especially the clothing industry, light engineering, transistor and assembly factories, and laundries. Texas Instruments, which employs women for the assembly of electrical components, finds that the average worker's normal production rate of 100 components per hour drops during the paramenstruum to 75 per hour.

Studies have shown that during the paramenstruum there is a deterioration of arm and hand steadiness, which is an adverse factor among those whose work demands manual dexterity. One podiatrist complained that during the paramenstruum her hands get stiff and she finds skilled movements difficult. "If I ever cut a patient, I'm sure it will be during those premenstrual days," she says. One wonders if the same ever applies to surgeons.

Absenteeism directly related to menstrual problems is generally caused by spasmodic dysmenorrhea, premenstrual migraine, and asthma. Other premenstrual symptoms are seldom a good enough reason to stay home, for, as one library assistant remarked, "You don't stay away from work merely because of your bad temper. Instead, you soldier on and cause chaos by misfiling, and you get yourself a bad name."

The influence of menstrual illness during working hours was demonstrated in a survey at a light-engineering factory in North London employing 3,500 women, and also in the branches of a department store employing 10,000 women. It showed that 45% of the 269 women surveyed who reported sick were in their paramenstruum. Dr. William Bickers and Maribelle Woods from the Medical College of Virginia noted as long ago as 1951 that 36% of women in their premenstrual week requested sedation during working hours.

Twenty years ago, a survey in four London hospitals showed that half of all emergency admissions of women to hospitals occurred during the premenstruum. These findings have since been confirmed worldwide. This figure was the same for medical emergencies (like coronaries and strokes), for surgical admissions (like colic and appendicitis), for infectious fevers, and for admissions to psychiatric wards. Admission for depression and suicides have been shown the world over to be the highest during the paramenstruum.

Accidents at work are another problem to industry, both the minor cuts and bruises, which are a waste of working time and are treated at the first aid station, and the serious ones, which require admission to the hospital. Research at the U.S. Center for Safety Education showed that the 48 hours before the onset of menstruation are the most dangerous ones, when most accidents occur. In Germany it was noted that apprentice tightrope walkers had the most accidents in the premenstruum. In restaurants it is recognized that the premenstrual clumsiness of waitresses accounts for an undue number of breakages.

Lowered mental ability during the paramenstruum also accounts for many unnecessary typing errors. More than one secretary has been referred for treatment when her boss could no longer put up with those few days every month when letters had to be repeatedly returned for retyping. Journalists, artists, and authors find this a problem too, lacking inspiration and waiting hopefully for a brainwave, which is more likely to come during the postmenstruum. Errors in billing, accounting, stocktaking, and filing take longer to correct than to make, and again the incidence of mistakes is highest during the paramenstruum. Premenstrual irritability may show itself in bad-tempered service by salespeople, receptionists, and waitresses, who are all in the public view. The problems of lowered judgment during the premenstruum must be considered by teachers, judges, and executives, who need to be on their guard against making hasty and wrong decisions. One teacher wrote with honesty, "Every month there are one or two days when I am simply not worth the salary my employers pay me."

Certain specialized occupations have their own particular hazards on premenstrual days. An example is the hoarseness that affects opera and other professional singers. One musical comedy star in the 1930s would, with devastating regularity, come into the theater once a month surrounded by a powerful aroma of garlic, which preceded her wherever she went. "You see," she would explain, "it's this sore throat again, and garlic is the only thing that saves my voice." Sure enough, 4 days later she would once again be in magnificent voice, but whether it was the garlic or her postmenstruum that was responsible is a matter of guesswork. For artists in the theater, premenstrual syndrome is a very real problem. One great impresario always attended rehearsals wearing a top hat and smoking a cigar. On one occasion his leading lady was making a fuss and was obviously in her premenstruum. The great man stood up in the center of the auditorium, ground his cigar to dust under his feet, and hurling his hat on the floor stamped on it, crying out, "Woman! I don't know why I employ you—you drive me to distraction!" There was a pause and in a changed voice he went on, "But when you are well, you're magnificent!"

One wonders how many so-called "prima donnas," with their reputation for throwing tantrums, were really only reacting to their premenstrual syndrome? For the members of the chorus, the showgirls, and ballet dancers, it is always a question of whether the stage manager has enough experience to realize their problem and help them over the difficult days. Their

symptoms of bloatedness and puffy eyes and skin are shared by
models and movie stars, who often have a clause in their con-
tracts forbidding filming during their paramenstruum. A lowered
sensitivity to taste is a handicap to cooks, who may over-flavor
the sauces and other foods. And we should remember the
woman astronaut, Russia's Valentina Tereshkova, who in 1973
had to be brought down after only 3 days in space when she
began to menstruate heavily in the zero gravity.

In Argentina, women are allowed under the Constitution
to take the necessary days off if they have menstrual problems.
In India, wives have long had the privilege of being excused
from housework, as it is believed that any food they prepare may
be spoiled.

The site of an individual's premenstrual symptoms may be
related to her work. In a study of premenstrual syndrome carried
out in a light-engineering factory about 20 women were interviewed in batches each day. Some days it was noted that the
predominant symptom was premenstrual backache, on other
days complaints of headaches were the most common. Later, it
became clear that all the women in any one batch came from
the same department and were doing the same kind of work.
Those who spent their working hours stooped over a workbench
were more likely to complain of backache, while those who sat
at a bench assembling small electrical parts, a task needing
considerable concentration, mostly complained of premenstrual
headaches.

Texas Instruments found that women had less menstrual
absenteeism when they worked from 2 P.M. to 10 P.M., compared
with the other shifts of 6 A.M. to 2 P.M. and 8:30 A.M. to 5:30 P.M.
Maybe this was because if they woke up feeling ill, they had
more time to take medicine and recover from their problems. It
is certainly worth considering for those who are given an option
to choose their own working hours. PMS sufferers usually cope
especially badly with night-shift work, which seems to be because the "diurnal clock," which regulates the sleep-wakefulness
cycle, is situated in the hypothalamus and easily disturbs the
menstrual clock. This is found to be a problem with nurses,
especially those in training, whose regulations demand a specified

period of night work. Night work often leads to upsets of the menstrual pattern and to depressive illness in sufferers of premenstrual syndrome.

Premenstrual syndrome can affect a woman's chances of getting employment, holding down a job, and receiving a promotion—or losing it unnecessarily. The problems of some sufferers are shown in the following excerpts from letters:

> "I cannot plan to go anywhere during these depressing times and I live in constant fear of losing my job, as I have to take time off each month with a real sick headache. My chances of promotion have been ruined because of this."

> "I recently gave up my job unnecessarily, and realized that it is ridiculous to let this condition ruin my whole life. Although I know the cause of my depressive feelings, I seem to be unable to think logically, and though I know I'll be fine again in a week, I get quite illogical and irrational at the same time."

> "I am 33 now and have suffered from premenstrual syndrome for the best part of my adult life. The symptoms are horrible depression, muddle-headedness, and feeling dead from the neck up. I recently took the totally unnecessary and very impulsive step of resigning from my job as an English teacher. Of course I took this drastic step just before my period. I am well-qualified and have been doing this now for 7 years. To all other people I appear cheerful, calm, and efficient, especially when a period is not close."

A different and very specialized hazard faced both male and female employees in the Ortho Pharmaceuticals oral contraceptive plant in Puerto Rico, where breast enlargement was found among the men and menstrual disorders among the women. This occurred despite the strict precautions taken in making the synthetic estrogens used in the contraceptives. These included hermetically sealed machines, air conditioners, respirators, and special protective clothing (even down to the underwear). The long-term effects of occupational exposure to estrogens are practically unknown, and there are no safety standards in force anywhere.

How can industry best cope with the financial burden caused by menstrual problems? Fortunately, many employers now have convenient restrooms where a woman can relax for a few hours, take something to ease her trouble, and return to continue her work. The availability of flextime, where each worker clocks herself in and out at times that suit her best, is a blessing to many women. They can accumulate a few hours reserve, so that when they are at their lowest they need not go to work at all.

But more is needed. Industry could tackle the situation better by educating staff, especially personnel managers and supervisors, to recognize and fully understand the problems so that they can deal with them better. For example, women can be assigned to less skilled jobs such as packing and stacking during their vulnerable days, rather than remaining on tasks that are more complex and harder to correct later, such as soldering or assembly.

Some enlightened organizations arrange talks on premenstrual syndrome for their workers and managers, and ensure that there are facilities for treatment locally. These treatment centers should be available either in hospitals or at places of employment.

14

Women at Leisure

Even when a woman is away from the office and the housework and just relaxing, the black cloud of once-a-month problems may still be with her. Which woman looking forward to a weekend of fun on a yacht or hiking in the mountains, on a bicycle or spelunking down in the caves, wants to be bothered with menstrual problems? Fortunately, something can be done for those women who are on the pill. They can be asked when they start their initial course, "Which day of the week would it be most convenient for you to menstruate?" As menstruation can be expected to start within 2 days of stopping the course, it is not very difficult to calculate which day to begin. Of course some women would find it more convenient to menstruate on the weekends, when their husbands can take over some domestic chores and care for the children.

SPORTS

The strenuous physical training and weight regulation demanded of top sportswomen often leads to delayed menarche, amenorrhea, infrequent and scanty menstruation, failure to ovulate, or infertility. These symptoms occur particularly in younger athletes, and those with a low body weight and low fat percentage, especially runners, gymnasts, and ballet dancers. When amenorrhea is present, menstruation, and sometimes also ovulation, may return when training is stopped because of vacations or injuries. Intensive physical activity can delay menarche if the activity is begun before puberty, and Frisch noted that among athletes who started training before their menarche the mean age of starting menstruation was 15.1 years, compared with athletes starting training after the menarche, who had an average menarcheal age of 12.8 years.

There is a positive correlation between these menstrual problems in athletes and the intensity of their training programs. Feicht and his colleagues showed that whereas only 6% of athletes running less than 10 miles weekly had amenorrhea, the figure rose to 43% for those running 70 miles or more weekly. Although superficially it may seem beneficial to be free of hazards of menstruation or fear of pregnancy, it is now becoming clear that the attendant lack of estrogen can result in brittle bones, as in postmenopausal women. So these young athletes become prone to stress fractures, especially of the metatarsal bones of the feet. Some studies on amenorrheic runners have shown that the bone mineral content was equivalent to that of the average 52-year-old woman, which suggests that they have an urgent need for calcium and estrogen supplementation to prevent premature osteoporosis.

What about the other sporting activities that women enjoy? Those who play tennis, golf, or racquetball may find that their performance deteriorates during the paramenstruum. It has been found that during this time arm and hand steadiness is impaired, sharpness of vision declines, and movement is slower because of extra weight and water retention. The menstrual influence on top sportswomen may be less obvious because they are able to maintain a steady standard with fewer fluctuations in performance. Since the mid-seventies, however, when research by the British Women's Amateur Athletic Association confirmed that top women athletes gave their best performances during their postmenstruum, trainers have started to do a little menstrual engineering, adjusting the time of menstruation so that the athletes do not have to rely entirely on Nature's roulette.

Drs. Moller-Neilsen and Hammar from Sweden confirmed

that women soccer players were more susceptible to injuries during their premenstruum and menstrual period than during the rest of the cycle, especially those with premenstrual symptoms of irritability, bloatedness, or breast discomfort. Fewer injuries occurred among those using oral contraceptives.

Dr. Ken Dyer of Adelaide, Australia, has produced some interesting figures showing that over the past 20 years women's top athletic performances have improved more than men's. This suggests that within the next three or four decades women could be running and swimming as well as men, certainly in the longer distance races. Women have determination and aggression, and are especially suited to prolonged exertion; there is the striking example of the Canadian, Cynthia Nicolas, who in the summer of 1977 set a new world record for crossing the English Channel twice in 19 hours 55 minutes, compared with the previous male record of 30 hours.

HOBBIES

Women have many hobbies, and it is difficult to cover them all. There are those who enjoy dressmaking, but know better than to cut a dress out of expensive material on the wrong day of the month in case they spoil it. Others hesitate to buy flowers at that time, as they find they cannot arrange them to their satisfaction. Artists often have difficulties or feel their inspiration is lost, and have to wait until their postmenstrual peak to resume creative activity.

Intellectual games may also be affected once a month, as the partner at bridge or the opponent at chess or scrabble may have discovered.

DRIVING HAZARDS

Driving is more necessary than recreational for most women, but for some it may be a sport or a social activity. A few may race cars, and many take motor trips, alone or with their families. In any case, there will be a menstrual handicap. A survey at four hospitals showed that half of all accident admissions of women occurred during their paramenstrual days. In fact, among those involved in an accident, the menstrual influence was equally present among the passengers, the passive participants, as among the drivers, the active participants. In the few seconds between a car climbing a curb and before it hits a wall an alert passenger may brace herself and cover her head for protection, but the passenger in her paramenstruum may be too slow to take even these elementary precautions.

Driving is a complicated task, requiring the coordination of many skills which are slower during the paramenstruum. Complicated and rapidly changing road situations demand quick reactions and good judgment, and if these are impaired, problems could result, like an increase in braking distance. Acuteness of hearing is dulled, so that a driver may not hear a warning siren. A decreased sharpness of vision and a lowered ability to judge shapes and sizes may cause a woman to lose her normal precision in parking and reversing. She may become impatient of the slow driver ahead, or of an elderly person crossing the road. She may overtake dangerously, or drive aggressively around a blind corner. She may fail to notice changing weather and light conditions, or alterations of the road surface. She may forget to fasten her safety belt, or follow other driving laws. Even as a pedestrian, she is more vulnerable in her paramenstruum, and may cross the road without the usual precautions. As a mother she may not be alert enough to protect her child from dangers on the road.

Having said all this, perhaps I should add that women are considered better risks than men by insurance companies. Though some women are at risk during the paramenstruum, they are much safer during the postmenstrual peak.

SHOPPING

The normal joys of a shopping spree may be ruined during the paramenstruum. A woman may become an indecisive, hesitant shopper who tries on all the shoes in the shop, finds they won't fit her swollen feet, and leaves empty-handed. She may buy totally inappropriate dresses, that don't fit and are the wrong color, and which she'll never wear. It is possible that her color sense and appreciation of shape and size deteriorate during this phase of the cycle. A few women even buy unnecessary and expensive items, like cars and jewelry. One woman in Arizona in two consecutive premenstruums bought two full-length mink coats, which she didn't need and could not really afford. One can't help feeling sorry for the man who wrote:

> "I know it's the wrong day of the month for my wife if I come home and find the kitchen loaded with fruit, anything up to 10 pounds of apples, bananas and oranges. I know she'll be in a terrible mood, and will ask me to put the children to bed . . . . But at other times she's the best wife in the world."

There is the problem of women shoplifters, who are caught during their paramenstruum. While it is possible that a few of them really are in a totally confused state and are unaware of what they are doing, others are habitual shoplifters who were caught because they were not quick enough or did not take their usual precautions.

ENTERTAINMENTS

Social entertainments may not be too successful during the paramenstruum. Cocktail parties too often require prolonged standing, which is no fun for those with water retention. As one woman put it:

> "I can always recognize fellow sufferers, as they also edge their way toward the walls to rest their legs."

Other problems related to this time of the month are described below:

> "My problem starts about 10 days before my period comes. I get uncontrollable fits of depression, which make me hit rock bottom. If I'm with a crowd of friends, I feel like I'm going to suffocate; it's a feeling that just sweeps over me and I want to run out, and I do run out."

"I often have to entertain for my husband. I am a good cook, even if I say so myself. I get an excellent meal ready, but when the first guest arrives I just burst into tears. It ruins my whole evening. I've learned to arrange the dates so that they come after my period, but then my period is bound to be late!"

Even the theater may not bring pleasure to everyone, as one sufferer from premenstrual depression recalled:

"I remember sitting in the theater with tears rolling down my cheeks, squeezing my hands and saying to myself, 'NO—I mustn't, this is a comedy—everyone else is laughing.' "

The problems of alcohol intoxication are increased during the paramenstruum, so that a woman can never really let herself go without getting into trouble. Some women can never take cannabis without suffering its worst effects, others can use it at most times of the month and enjoy the experience. However, if they smoke it during the paramenstruum they may develop delusions or hallucinations.

Some women have an uncontrollable urge to gamble during the premenstruum, whether it is on horses, cards, or bingo. One of my patients is addicted to slot machines. Some days she is just spellbound by them, and cannot stop. Now that she realizes the cause of her habit, she tries to go out without any money at those times of the month.

VACATIONS

Vacations are not always as much fun as anticipated, in fact, sometimes they are complete disasters. Flights may be delayed, so that eating schedules are completely thrown off. Women should bear this in mind when packing their carry-on luggage, and keep a supply of emergency rations with them. Remember that food is not served on the plane immediately after departure, or when the plane is circling its destination for what seems like hours before receiving permission to land. Hotels in other countries may have fixed hours for meals with no arrangements for mid-morning, mid-afternoon, or late-night snacks.

Avoid night travel as much as possible, as this disturbs the day/night rhythm center in the hypothalamus, which is close to the menstrual controlling center. PMS sufferers are likely to have trouble with jet lag for the same reason. After a long flight, they should go straight to bed regardless of the time of day, avoiding the temptation to do some quick sightseeing or to chat with friends. A few hours rest will do wonders to prevent the terrible lethargy that results from jet lag and can last for days.

15

Premenstrual Syndrome Goes to Court

In a surprising coincidence, two women in different English cities appeared in court on consecutive days, each charged with murder. Both had their charges reduced to manslaughter on grounds of diminished responsibility by reason of premenstrual syndrome. Although the circumstances of the two offenses differed, the evidence in each case led to the same conclusion: the defendant was suffering from severe PMS. Both cases had been very carefully researched, and presented indisputable evidence of long-standing, bizarre, cyclical behavior occurring in the premenstruum, with normalcy of behavior in the postmenstruum. It is important to keep in mind that these were two extreme and exceptional cases. Not all sufferers of premenstrual syndrome are potential murderers, nor do all female murderers suffer from premenstrual syndrome. The International Symposium on Premenstrual, Postpartum, and Menopausal Mood Disorders held at Kiawah Island, South Carolina, in 1987, confirmed that the number of cases of severe premenstrual syndrome of the type described in these legal defenses and sensationalized by the press is extremely small.

This legal ruling recognizing premenstrual syndrome places a new responsibility on the medical professions. It is now their duty to ensure that the plea of premenstrual syndrome will not be abused, and that any such plea adheres to the strict definition. This requires the diagnosis of PMS to be substantiated with evidence in every case and the condition must respond to treatment. There must be evidence of recurrent symptoms; or earlier episodes of a similar loss of control, confusion, or amnesia; or violence in previous cycles or at monthly intervals. Women facing charges of shoplifting are often referred to me by their lawyers, who hope to use premenstrual syndrome as a defense. I first give them the definition of premenstrual syndrome and then ask "What did you steal in the last 2 months, before your menstruation?" This is usually enough of a shock, and most of them leave the consulting room hurriedly, muttering, "But this really is my first offense . . . ."

FACTUAL EVIDENCE IS REQUIRED

The necessary evidence, if it is there, may be found in diaries, medical records, police files, or prison documents. These often give the precise dates of marital quarrels, physical violence, previous suicide attempts, and other serious incidents. One woman accused of manslaughter had 30 previous convictions, occurring at cycles of 29.04 ± 1.47 days. The documents also showed that while in prison she had made attempts at drowning and strangling herself, escaping, slashing her wrists, smashing windows, and setting fire to the bed in her cell. These incidents had been carefully recorded by prison officers and were found to have occurred at intervals of 29.55 ± 1.45 days. Thus, the diagnosis did not rely on the woman's memory. Prison records also showed that she had been described as "pleasant and cooperative, but at times loses her senses and can be quite impulsive," which suggests that destructive symptoms were completely absent after menstruation.

An 18-year-old ballet dancer who was accused of arson successfully pleaded premenstrual syndrome as a mitigating factor, and was released on probation. She had an excellent school record, and her behavior had always been exemplary until she started menstruating. After that she appeared to change in character, and had severe episodes of unusual and unexplained behavior. One day she suddenly went into her bedroom and shaved off her blonde hair and eyebrows; another time, she ran away from home and was later returned by the police, having been found drunk and disorderly; once she burned the bedroom curtains; another time she overdosed on pain relievers and alcohol and was hospitalized for a night; finally, she set fire to her father's house and was sent to prison. While in prison she tried to set fire to the bed in her cell. On another occasion she attempted to strangle herself by tying one end of a sheet around her neck and the other end to the top of the window.

It was her father who noticed from his diaries that his daughter's problems occurred about once a month. He was advised to produce proof that would show the precise dates on which the different events occurred. He did this by searching through the doctor's and hospital's files, and by checking the dates of insurance claims for the burned curtains, the date on the check with which he bought his daughter a new wig, and the precise dates on which she misbehaved while in prison. The many occurrences were clearly shown to be coming in regular monthly cycles. Ultimately, the girl received progesterone treatment and is now a successful executive.

A similar story is the one of an unemployed girl who harassed the police with unnecessary emergency phone calls. She had earlier been sent to a reform school for the same offense, but after being released she persisted with the calls and was imprisoned. Again, her father was the one who noticed that the problems occurred every month, and told the lawyer. In her case the calls represented a cry for help, akin to other women whose cry for attention might be a suicide attempt or self-mutilation. She, too, responded to progesterone and was released on probation. However, after she left prison the progesterone was not continued, and she again began making unnecessary police phone calls. This time no mercy was shown, and she served a 2-year sentence. That was 6 years ago; today, on progesterone treatment, her life has changed and she is working with the disabled, is happily married, and has one son.

In 1977 a 46-year-old part-time social worker was charged

with shoplifting. In court she produced her diary, showing the days of confusion each month when she refused to leave the house. It showed that she had arranged her days at work accordingly. Her husband had recognized the cyclical symptoms, and described how she would return from shopping with dog food although they had no pets, or a child's ski outfit although their own children were now grown. Together the husband and wife had marked in the diary the days on which trouble might occur. All was well until a co-worker caught the flu and the social worker agreed to alter her working days. The case was dismissed. She has since received progesterone treatment and has been free from these lapses of concentration and confusion.

These represent genuine cases of criminal behavior resulting from a hormonal disease that responds to treatment. These women deserve to be freed, for they cannot be held responsible for their unexpected loss of control. However, the genuine cases are few and far between, and it is important to ensure that premenstrual syndrome is not made a universal defense. Cases have already occurred in Britain where this has been tried. A woman on her first charge of shoplifting cannot claim premenstrual syndrome as a defense without evidence that this is a recurring problem. And the mere coincidence of two car crashes or two speeding offenses occurring in the premenstruum cannot be considered sufficient evidence.

For a correct diagnosis of premenstrual syndrome, the precise dates of menstruation and of the alleged crime are necessary. Yet a clerk in a travel agency, accused of stealing travelers' checks worth $1,000 from her employer on some unknown date between August 1980 and April 1981, pleaded premenstrual syndrome. Not surprisingly, the plea failed and a jail sentence was imposed.

When a woman pleads PMS in her defense, the public still has a right to be protected by the knowledge that the defendant is receiving progesterone treatment and is unlikely to be a further danger. Because PMS is a recurrent illness, the woman, if not treated, is liable to repeat the offense. However, PMS should not be used as a defense if the woman is likely to repeat her offense, be it murder, assault, damage to property, or shoplifting. At an appeals trial in Britain, premenstrual syndrome was rejected as a defense in a case of murder, although it still stands as a "factor causing diminished responsibility" in capital charges, and as "a mitigating factor" in lesser charges.

CHARACTERISTICS OF PMS OFFENSES

There are certain characteristics of the offenses committed by sufferers of PMS which may be easily recognized:

1) The woman acts alone without an accomplice

2) The offense is not premeditated, and usually comes as a surprise even to those whom she was with shortly before the event

3) The action is without clear motive, such as setting fire to an unknown person's property

4) There may be no attempt to escape detection. A woman may randomly throw a brick in a shop window and then telephone the police herself and await her arrest

5) The action may be a *cri de coeur*, as with the girl who repeatedly makes emergency 911 calls. This is similar to parasuicide.

Among the more frequent symptoms of premenstrual syndrome that may result in criminal acts are a sudden and momentary surge of uncontrollable emotion resulting in violence, confusion or amnesia, alcoholism, nymphomania, and attention-seeking episodes that represent cries for help. The resulting actions may cover a full range of criminal offenses such as actual violence, damage to property, theft, and disorderly behavior.

IDENTIFYING PMS OFFENDERS

Sufferers of premenstrual syndrome characteristically have pain-free menstruation. The shoplifter who claimed her period pains were so severe that she was under the influence of pain-relieving drugs at the time of her offenses, was suffering from spasmodic dysmenorrhea and not from premenstrual syndrome.

A full medical history will reveal information that can confirm or disprove the diagnosis. The onset of premenstrual syndrome and the occasions of increased severity always occur at times of hormonal upheaval, such as puberty, during or after taking the pill, or after amenorrhea, pregnancy, or sterilization. The women involved have side effects on the pill, and their pregnancy may be complicated by pre-eclampsia or postnatal depression. During the premenstruum they have difficulty in tolerating long intervals without food (over 5 hours daytime or 13 hours overnight), and they become easily intoxicated by alcohol while in the premenstruum.

A 32-year-old Essex housewife was accused of infanticide, having drowned her second daughter and then overdosed herself. She started menstruating in the intensive care unit and mention of premenstrual syndrome was noted in her previous medical records. She had developed migraine and hypertension on the pill, for which she was admitted for observation to the London Hospital. Her first pregnancy was complicated by pre-eclampsia, and after her second pregnancy she developed postnatal depression requiring psychiatric attention. The incident occurred about 5:30 P.M., and she had had no food since her 8:30 A.M. breakfast. The court accepted the several diagnostic pointers indicating PMS, and she was released on probation and treatment.

Among women with PMS, increased libido is occasionally noticed in the premenstruum, a fact recorded by Israel back in 1938. As mentioned before, this urge may be responsible for adolescent girls running away from home. These girls can be helped, and their criminal career abruptly ended with hormone therapy.

Some women who suffer greatly from premenstrual syndrome are needlessly incarcerated. They are deserving of our sympathy, and justice will not be served until all true sufferers of premenstrual syndrome are properly diagnosed and treated. The road to rehabilitation after a prison sentence is long and hard. The interests of all women will be served best by increasing our diagnostic capacity, enabling us to distinguish the few genuine sufferers from the many malingerers, whose claims of premenstrual syndrome can never be substantiated. Further information on this subject is contained in my book, *Premenstrual Syndrome Goes to Court* (Peter Andrew Publishing, Droitwich, U.K.).

16

The Hormonal Control

Some scientists believe that the body is governed by bio-rhythms, which include a physical rhythm of 23 days, a sensitivity or emotional rhythm of 28 days, and an intellectual rhythm of 33 days. These body cycles are not affected by life events and repeat themselves without change so that they can be charted for any individual if the hour and date of birth is known. The menstrual cycle should not be associated with these biorhythms in any way; it is completely different. No matter how precisely you can pinpoint your hour and date of birth, it will not enable you or anyone else to work out when your menstrual cycle will begin, what its length will be, or anything at all about your patterns of ovulation and menstruation.

The menstrual cycle does not begin at birth. It is interrupted by pregnancy and breastfeeding, and it is altered by life events such as illnesses, examinations, bereavement, happy times, sad events, and changes in environment. Menstrual patterns show endless variations in duration of flow and quantity of blood lost, as well as in the length of cycle.

When discussing the menstrual cycle it is convenient to consider a 28-day cycle. It makes things simpler and is easier when discussing the various changes that occur, such as ovulation on the fourteenth day. But we should not forget that women are all individuals and do not fit neatly into pigeonholes. Sometimes I am asked, "What is the right length of the menstrual cycle?" One might as well ask, "What is the right height for a woman?" Individuals differ: there are healthy, normal women who menstruate every 21 days, and those at the other extreme who menstruate on average every 36 days. Both are normal, with fully effective reproductive systems. The cycle of 28 days is an approximate average for all women all over the world. Chiazze and his colleagues found that only 62% of women aged 15–19 years had a menstrual cycle between 25 and 31 days, with the proportion gradually increasing with age, so that 86% of those aged 35–39 years had an *almost* conventional cycle.

It is said that Dr. Pinkus, the father of the pill, decided over a cup of tea with the British endocrinologist Peter Bishop that 28 days would be a convenient time interval to allow withdrawal bleeding to occur in women on the pill. So it is that today there are millions of women with man-made cycles of 28 days. But they could just as easily have decided on 24 days or 30 days.

When women are asked the length of their cycle, they frequently reply, "Oh, I'm always late," meaning it is longer than 28 days, or, "I'm quite regular," meaning "I never get worried, because I'm never over 28 days." Incidentally, the days of a cycle should always be counted from the first day of menstruation until the first day of the next menstruation. Confusion sometimes occurs because women count from the end of one period until the beginning of the next, counting only the days they are not bleeding.

The duration of the menstrual flow also varies from cycle to cycle and from individual to individual. It may be as short as 2 days or go on as long as 8 days, and doctors would still consider it normal and know that these women would be able to have children if they so desired. The quantity of the menstrual flow or blood loss is equally variable. Few people are likely to see another person's flow, so there is bound to be considerable exaggeration in both directions. Some women will say, "I had a really good period," by which they might mean the loss was bright red; many women object to the scanty dark red, brown, or black loss that sometimes comes with the pill. It is helpful to realize that menstrual bleeding comes from the minute blood vessels in the lining of the womb and not from any big blood vessels, so that if bleeding continued for a long time it might cause anemia but one can never actually bleed to death as one could from a wound.

The type of flow is also different in different women. Some start with a heavy loss that continues for a few days and then stops abruptly. Others start more gradually, with 1 or 2 days of scanty loss before the full flow, and then end either abruptly or gradually over a few days. All these types are normal, but the symptoms of premenstrual syndrome do not end until the full menstrual flow, so that some women may have problems during the first few days of menstruation.

THE MENSTRUAL CONTROLLING CENTER

In the opening chapter the menstrual cycle was broken down into seven 4-day phases of hormone activity. Each hormone change is carefully monitored by the menstrual controlling center, often referred to as the "menstrual clock." This is not situated in the womb where the action takes place but at a distance from it, low in the brain, in a part known as the "hypothalamus." (See Figure 20.) The hypothalamus itself controls or orchestrates many other functions and centers, among them the centers for the control of water balance, appetite, weight, mood, and the day/night rhythm. Thus, if any one of these is upset it will tend to affect the others. The diagram in Figure 21 shows the proximity of these centers. This explains why, when the menstrual cycle is disturbed or altered (such as by taking the pill), it can upset the weight balance, the water balance, and the mood centers, causing weight-gain, water retention, and depression. If the appetite is drastically curtailed, as in anorexia nervosa, the menstrual cycle will stop and depression will develop. Depressive illnesses, in turn, are likely to cause an alteration in menstrual patterns, resulting either in excessive bleeding, as in the "weeping womb," or a break in

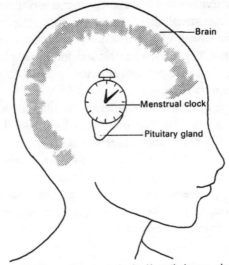

It is at the base of the brain in the Hypothalamus, above the Pituitary gland.

Figure 20 Position of the menstrual clock

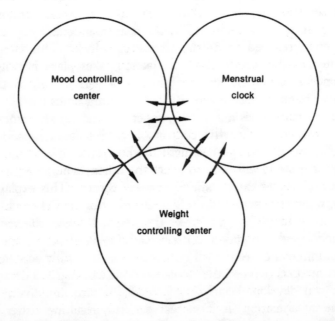

Figure 21 Diagram of controlling centers in the hypothalamus

menstruation. They can also cause alterations in weight, either a gain or a loss.

The diurnal controlling center, which is concerned with sleep rhythms, is also situated in the hypothalamus, close to the menstrual clock. Those with a sensitive menstrual clock are likely to be easily upset by night-shift work, and experience severe jet lag after long flights.

MENSTRUAL CLOCK

The menstrual clock, which is the control center of the menstrual cycle, is responsible for the smooth and effective operation of a woman's marvelous reproductive system. Situated in the hypothalamus, it has two hormones that it uses for this purpose. Hormones are chemical messengers with their own individual structure; they travel in the bloodstream and are designed to act on a particular target organ. The two hormones that serve the menstrual clock have rather grand-sounding names: Follicle Stimulating Hormone Releasing Hormone (FSHRH) and Luteinising Hormone Releasing Hormone (LHRH). Their target is the pituitary gland, situated next to the hypothalamus at the base of the brain. These two releasing hormones stimulate the pituitary gland to produce two other menstrual hormones mentioned earlier: Follicle Stimulating Hormone (FSH) and Luteinising Hormone (LH), thus boosting the hormone output. (See Figure 22.)

The pituitary gland sends out a variety of different hormones that control, among other things, growth, pigmentation, lactation, thyroid function, and adrenalin and insulin output. In short, it has a finger in every pie. But what concerns us now are the two pituitary hormones, FSH and LH, which act on the ovaries. FSH acts on the ovaries to stimulate the formation of follicles, tiny microscopic rings of cells within which lies an immature ovum or egg cell. As the follicles develop, specialized cells produce estrogen, yet another hormone, which is released into the blood stream. Estrogen builds up the lining of the womb to replace the one that was shed at the last menstruation. It also has another important function: before ovulation it thins

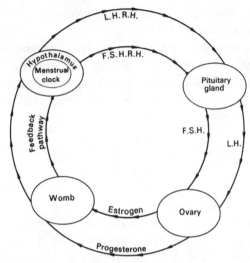

Figure 22 Menstrual hormonal pathways

the cervical mucus, or natural vaginal discharge, to assist the sperm entering the womb in their search for the egg cell, which needs to be fertilized for pregnancy to occur. Estrogen is also responsible, at puberty, for the development of the secondary sex characteristics: breast development, hair growth, and the rounded female physique.

At mid-cycle a sudden surge of the other pituitary hormone, luteinising hormone, causes the ripened follicle to burst and discharge its egg cell, a process known as "ovulation." Further stimulation by LH causes new cells to form at the site of the burst follicle, and these cells produce the other menstrual hormone, progesterone. Progesterone is secreted in spurts, and after ovulation it passes in the blood stream to its target organ, the womb. The levels of these hormones during a normal menstrual cycle are shown in Figure 1, page 13.

After the lining of the womb has been rebuilt under the influence of estrogen, it is converted by progesterone into a soft, spongy tissue that is ready for the embedding of a fertilized egg. Thus progesterone is needed *after* ovulation, when the initial repair work on the lining of the womb has already taken place. Progesterone is also responsible for making the fallopian tubes contract more forcefully but less frequently, so that the egg cell may be swept along to the womb. Progesterone also changes the vaginal discharge from a thin watery, fluid in which sperm can move freely into a thick, sticky mucus, which prevents further sperm from entering the womb. The presence of progesterone raises the body temperature again, in preparation for a possible pregnancy.

Another control of the menstrual clock is prolactin, a hormone produced by the anterior pituitary gland which is involved in the progesterone feedback mechanism. If too much prolactin is produced the progesterone feedback pathway is interrupted.

Nature has devised a magnificent system in our reproductive process, complete with a highly efficient communication network between the hypothalamus, pituitary, ovary, and womb, which is called the "feedback pathway." This ensures that the higher centers are kept fully informed of the progress in the ovaries and the womb (see Figure 22) and can adjust the level of hormones accordingly. For instance, if conception occurs, the hormonal output is altered within hours.

OVULATION

Most women know when ovulation occurs because they experience a slight discomfort for about an hour in one side of the lower abdomen. At the same time, they may notice that their normal vaginal discharge changes from a thin fluid to a thick, sticky mucus. Some women develop a migraine at that time, or tend to be irritable, while for the more unfortunate this may herald the onset of premenstrual syndrome. Sometimes, when the migraine or irritability at ovulation is severe, women have difficulty in becoming pregnant because they avoid intercourse on the very days that they are most likely to conceive.

If a woman records her temperature carefully for 2 minutes every morning before getting out of bed, she may be able to tell if she is ovulating, and also whether she has sufficient progesterone. In Figure 23 a few temperature charts are shown. *Teresa* is normal: ovulation occurred as shown by the sudden dip and

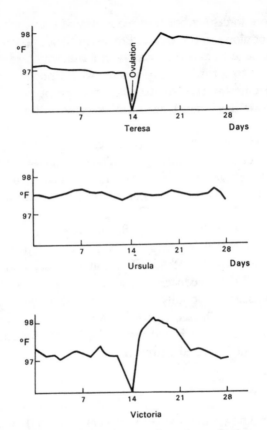

Figure 23 Temperature charts taken through the menstrual cycle

subsequent rise in temperature until the start of menstruation. *Ursula*'s chart is very steady and all on the same level, with no evidence of ovulation; it is known as an "anovular chart." *Victoria*'s chart does show ovulation and a rise in temperature, but this rise is not maintained, suggesting that she has insufficient progesterone. Not all temperature charts are reliable, however; ovulation can occur even with a chart like Ursula's.

The exact time of ovulation can be determined in several ways: by the change from a thin discharge to thick, sticky mucus; from a daily temperature chart; using tests showing the time of the peak of LH in the blood; and by direct inspection of

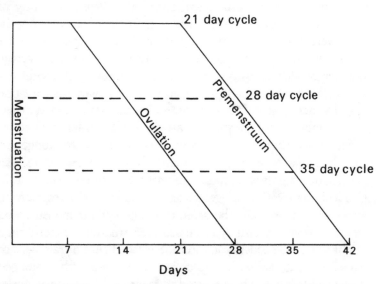

Figure 24 Timing of ovulation with different lengths of cycles

the ovary, either at the time of an abdominal operation or by laparascopy, in which a minute periscope is inserted through the abdominal wall. The most reliable method, however, is serial ultrasound scans of the ovaries. Ovulation occurs 12–14 days before the onset of menstruation, so it is only correct to talk about ovulation at mid-cycle in a woman whose cycle averages 28 days. In those who have a longer cycle, ovulation occurs after mid-cycle, as shown in Figure 24. In women with a 35-day cycle, ovulation is likely to occur about day 21; in those with a cycle of 21 days, it is more likely to occur about day 10.

EMOTIONAL UPSET OF MENSTRUATION

The menstrual clock is a very delicate mechanism, requiring a precise hormone balance to ensure trouble-free menstruation. It is easily upset by stresses of all kinds, both happy events such as weddings, holidays, and promotions, and unpleasant events like examinations, bereavements, and financial or marital problems.

The extent to which emotions can affect the timing of menstruation was shown in a study of 91 boarding school girls, who were taking their tenth-grade high school exams in the second week of June. Each day before the exams the average number of girls menstruating was 16, but during the vital examination week as many as 36 girls were menstruating on one day. In fact, just under half showed some alteration in their normal menstrual pattern. In some the cycle was lengthened, in others it was shortened. In many, menstruation lasted longer, so that it spread over into examination week. There were also about a dozen girls who missed menstruation entirely that month. Clinical observation suggests that an individual's reaction to stress tends to remain the same throughout their menstruating years, so that the girls who missed menstruation at exam time might also stop suddenly in later life if faced with a traumatic or stressful event. Similarly, the ones who reacted with prolonged menstrual loss could be expected to react in the same way under severe stress in later life.

One letter writer asked:

> "Since my husband was killed in a sailing accident last year my periods have been very irregular and much heavier. I am now over the loss, have a new job, and only get depressed before a period. Is this anything to worry about?"

The short answer is: No. A horrible shock like this is bound to be felt by the hypothalamus, which in turn will temporarily upset the normal menstrual pattern. As the woman appears to be adjusting her life to the tragedy, it is likely that her menstruation will gradually return to its old pattern.

MENSTRUAL SYNCHRONY

Another point to be considered with regard to the timing of menstruation is called "menstrual synchrony," which is when a number of women's menstruations occur together. This happens among women who live close together in closed communities like communes, prisons, convents, college campuses, and school dormitories. Especially if they share common emotional experiences, such as examinations and end-of-school excitement, their menstruation gradually becomes synchronized. This in turn raises fresh problems, because if more than one woman is suffering from premenstrual tension, trouble is inevitable. It is often necessary, for example, to move women prisoners from one cell to another before such synchronization occurs.

Menstrual synchrony is frequently noticed in mothers and daughters. If a daughter is brought to the doctor by her mother and is unable to remember the date of her last menstruation, chances are that the mother will reply and then add, "our dates always come together." Similarly, menstruation tends to coincide in lesbians. The mechanism of this synchronization is not clear, but it has been suggested that it may be related to sensitive body odors or pheromones.

The potency of these menstrual hormones is almost unbelievable. The powder a woman uses to cover the tip of her nose weighs many times more than the total amount of female hormones in her bloodstream. Yet they cause the sex organs and breasts to grow to mature size, and they bring about changes in bone structure and fat distribution that mold her figure into feminine contours and bring her to the peak of womanhood and motherhood.

SEX HORMONE BINDING GLOBULIN

Hormones are chemical messengers, made in one organ and having their action on some other organ or tissue. Sex hormones can be attached, or bound, in the blood to a minute protein molecule called "globulin." The capacity of this sex hormone binding globulin (SHBG) to bind to dihydrotestosterone, another hormone, is measured in the SHBG blood test that was mentioned in Chapter 3 as a diagnostic aid for premenstrual syndrome. Just how this fits into the jigsaw puzzle of premenstrual syndrome is not yet known. Why is the SHBG low in women with premenstrual syndrome? Why does the level of SHBG rise when progesterone is administered to sufferers of premenstrual syndrome? Again, why does the SHBG fall when progestogens are administered? These are among the many riddles that are still awaiting solution as we try to increase our understanding of premenstrual syndrome.

HORMONE RECEPTORS

When a hormone has been conveyed in the blood to the tissue where its action is required, it is transported into the cell nucleus by means of a hormone receptor. Hormone receptors are situated within the tissue cells; they key onto a single molecule of their special hormone and convey it through the cell substance and the nuclear wall into the nucleus, where the hormone is converted and used. Hormone receptors are very specific and will only transport the special hormone for which they are made, be it thyroid, cortisone, estrogen, or progesterone.

Progesterone receptors are present in the lining of the womb, where their presence is understandable, but it is their distribution in other parts of the body that is of special interest. These are tissues that utilize progesterone in the luteal phase (the days from ovulation to menstruation), although the precise purpose of progesterone within these cells is not fully known. Progesterone receptors are found in many places in the body, with the largest concentration in the limbic area of the midbrain, a part that animal biologists refer to as the "area of rage and violence." It seems possible that an insufficiency of progesterone in the midbrain receptors may be responsible for premenstrual tension. Progesterone receptors are also found in the nasopharyngeal passages and lungs and in the eyes, breasts, and liver. Many other premenstrual symptoms occur in just these areas: rhinitis, sinusitis, laryngitis, and asthma in the nasopharyngeal passages and lungs; conjunctivitis, styes, uveitis, and glaucoma in the eyes; and mastitis in the breasts. This widespread distribution of progesterone receptors in target cells explains the numerous different symptoms of premenstrual syndrome.

When progesterone is taken by mouth, it passes to the liver, the site of numerous progesterone receptors, where it is broken down and used, instead of being transported in the blood to the other target sites referred to in the previous paragraph, which contain progesterone receptors and where the progesterone is required. With oral progesterone, therefore, the concentration of progesterone reaching the systemic blood and the brain is very low.

There are no hormone receptors for the man-made progestogen drugs. They may force themselves into testosterone receptors or progesterone receptors, but they do not do this equally well in all the progesterone receptor sites in the body.

With increasing knowledge has come the realization that hormones do not have a single action but act on many systems. One has only to think of the widespread effects of an excess of thyroid hormone, or of the deficiency of insulin that occurs in diabetes. Estrogen, in addition to its action on the reproductive system, is also involved in cholesterol balance, bone metabolism, blood circulation, and skin elasticity.

PROGESTERONE

Irene Elias, in *The Female Animal*, reminds us that progesterone is the oldest steroid, being some 500 million years old on the evolutionary scale. It is present in all vertebrates, which includes frogs, snakes, birds, and fishes. Of course not all vertebrates menstruate, nor do they require progesterone for reproduction, but in the lower vertebrates progesterone is involved in glucose metabolism and the development of intelligence. The role of progesterone in the enhancement of intelligence has also been demonstrated in my surveys of 1968 and 1976, which showed that 32% of children whose mothers received progesterone during pregnancy went on to a university, compared with 6% of controls; 6% is also the national average in Britain. In humans, progesterone is present in the adrenals in men, women, and children, and is converted into other steroid hormones, such as cortisone, estrogen, and testosterone.

PROGESTERONE RECEPTORS

The study of the characteristics of progesterone receptors has had to rely on animal studies, because there have been no volunteers for brain biopsies from among normal women or from premenstrual syndrome sufferers. However, we have learned from the molecular biologists that, being a steroid, molecules of progesterone can pass through the cell wall into the substance of the cell. Once there the molecules need to combine with progesterone receptors to form a "hormone-receptor complex" in order to be transported into the nucleus and DNA, where they can be broken down and used.

Blaustein has demonstrated the ability of progesterone receptors to accept an initial dose of progesterone, but subsequent doses need to be some 40 times the original dose before they can form a hormone-receptor complex. No explanation has been given yet for this surprising progesterone receptor requirement. However, it is known that during pregnancy the blood progesterone level rises to almost 40 times the peak level found in the luteal phase of the menstrual cycle. (See Figure 25.) This massive increase in progesterone is produced by the placenta within the womb, and is essentially for the benefit of the fetus. Nevertheless, it is known that women with premenstrual syndrome are entirely free from their premenstrual symptoms during the latter half of pregnancy, and indeed many blossom at this time, which would seem to indicate that they are sharing this massive increase in progesterone production with the fetus.

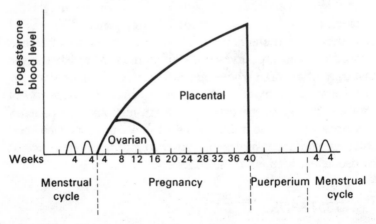

Figure 25 Levels of progesterone during the menstrual cycle and pregnancy

Could it be that there is a central control system that, while ensuring there is sufficient progesterone for the developing fetus, controls the distribution of any surplus to the mother? If this control system failed to return to a normal pre-pregnancy state, it might account for the resurgence of premenstrual symptoms or the development of postnatal depression immediately after the delivery of the placenta, and also explain why premenstrual syndrome so frequently begins, or increases in severity, after a pregnancy, for there might be insufficient progesterone to stimulate the progesterone receptors. It would also explain the failure of the low doses of progesterone used in double-blind clinical trials, which have never shown the beneficial effect of progesterone.

There is no evidence of any such high requirement of estrogen molecules by estrogen receptors, and so the doses of estrogen used in hormone replacement therapy are physiological, being the normal functioning level of about 1 or 2 milligrams daily.

Another important characteristic of progesterone receptors demonstrated by Nock is that they cannot convey molecules of progesterone to the nucleus of cells in the presence of adrenalin.

BLOOD SUGAR LEVELS

Progesterone also plays a part in the regulation of the blood sugar (or blood glucose) level. There are two regulating mechanisms, an upper and a lower, that ensure that the blood sugar always remains close to the optimum level. These prevent the blood sugar level from becoming too high (hyperglycemia), or too low (hypoglycemia), both of which may cause loss of consciousness or death. (See Figure 26.) Essentially, the blood sugar level is maintained by eating carbohydrates, the energy-giving foods that include starches (flour, potatoes, oats, rye, and rice) and sugars. Eating sugars causes a rapid rise and rapid drop in blood sugar level, whereas eating starches brings a more gradual and sustained rise and a slower fall. If a large quantity of carbohydrates is eaten at one time, the upper regulating mechanism is brought into play. There is a surge of insulin, and a valve opens that releases the extra sugar into the urine (renal threshold). On the other hand, if there is a long interval without food and the blood sugar level drops very low, it may activate the lower regulating mechanism and cause a sudden outpouring of adrenalin. This adrenalin mobilizes some of the sugar stored in other cells of the body and passes it into the blood, so that the blood sugar level is again restored to the optimum level. (See Figure 26.) This is achieved by special hormone receptors for the blood sugar known as glucocorticoid receptors. However, when sugar is taken from the cells, they fill up with water, and this is responsible for water retention, bloatedness, and weight-gain, which is such a common feature of premenstrual syndrome.

When a woman eats a meal, such as a breakfast of eggs and toast, the blood sugar level rises immediately and then falls gradually over the next 4 or 5 hours. If she eats again after 3 or

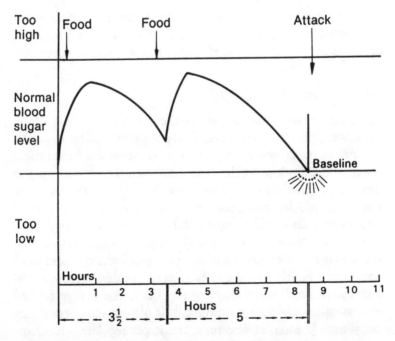

Figure 26 Effect of food on blood sugar levels

4 hours, the blood sugar will again rise immediately and then fall slowly. However, if she does not take any more food for a long interval the blood sugar will continue to drop until it reaches the lower regulating mechanism or baseline, causing an outpouring of adrenalin.

Adrenalin is the hormone that mobilizes the body's "fright, fight, and flight" response, and a sudden outpouring of adrenalin could trigger attacks of irritability, migraine, panic, or epilepsy in some women. In others, it might cause feelings of being weak, shivery, and faint, or bring on palpitations. On the other hand, there are also those fortunate individuals who can manage long fasts, as they are unaware when their blood sugar baseline has been reached and they get renewed energy from their own sugar stores.

Many women will have noticed that they can easily diet and go 5 hours without food after menstruation, but they have marked food cravings before menstruation. Giving progesterone

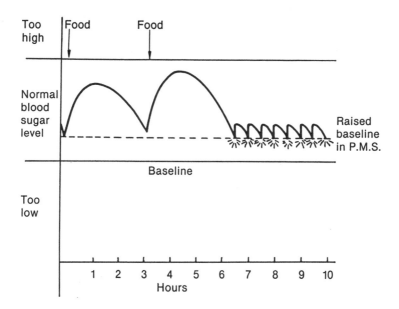

Figure 27 Effect of food on blood sugar levels in women with premenstrual syndrome

helps to correct this premenstrual alteration of the blood sugar level.

Progesterone is involved in the lower regulating mechanism and if, before menstruation, there is insufficient progesterone, the baseline is raised. (See Figure 27.) This means that women with premenstrual syndrome will tend to reach the level at which the lower regulating mechanism comes into action at an earlier stage. In practice this is usually about 3 hours after the ingestion of starchy food, so women are advised to eat small portions of starchy food every 3 hours. Men, on the other hand, can usually go longer without replenishment, as their lower regulating mechanism is set at a different level.

The attacks of fainting, panic, crying, irritability, or headache brought on by fasting and a resulting drop in blood sugar level are sometimes erroneously called "hypoglycemic attacks." Doctors do not like that usage as the term "hypoglycemic" is reserved for those whose blood sugar stays below the baseline and below the normal blood sugar level. In normal women, Nature's fail-safe control prevents hypoglycemia from occurring.

17

🕭

What Goes Wrong?

THE CAUSE OF PREMENSTRUAL SYNDROME

The cause of premenstrual syndrome is a subject most research workers avoid. Even medical journals prefer publishing failed treatment trials to discussing what goes wrong to cause premenstrual syndrome. Any theory about its origin must explain all that is known about it. This includes:

1) It only occurs in women during the reproductive years

2) Symptoms are present in the premenstruum and absent in the postmenstruum

3) Symptoms are absent during the second half of pregnancy, but severe attacks may occur after delivery

4) Symptoms start at puberty, after a pregnancy, after a spell of amenorrhea, after stopping the pill, and after sterilization and hysterectomy and/or oophorectomy. These are all times when the menstrual controlling center in the brain has been upset

5) Premenstrual syndrome can occur in both ovular and

anovular cycles, and can be present in the year or two before menstruation starts and after it ends

6) The 150 symptoms that may occur in premenstrual syndrome can also occur in men, children, and post-menopausal women. Also, there are more somatic than psychological symptoms

7) Women with premenstrual syndrome have difficulty tolerating long intervals without food and are liable to binges, especially on sweets

8) Symptoms increase at times of stress and after a long interval without food

9) There is a good response to systemic progesterone if it is given in high doses, although double-blind control-led trials of low dose progesterone suggest progesterone is no better than placebos

10) Studies have shown that premenstrual syndrome is not related to blood levels of progesterone, estrogen, FSH, LH, aldosterone, prolactin, or serotonin.

PROGESTERONE RECEPTORS ARE THE KEY

Recent work in molecular biochemistry has revealed the importance of progesterone receptors in the body's utilization of the progesterone circulating in the body, and an understanding of the characteristics of progesterone receptors and glucocorticoid receptors (see page 150) has provided an explanation for all the facts listed above. This suggests that progesterone receptors are the missing link in our understanding of what goes wrong in premenstrual syndrome: either there are not enough proges-terone receptors to transport the molecules of progesterone into the nucleus, or the ability of the receptors is inhibited by adrenalin or some other unknown factor.

This new knowledge suggests that premenstrual syndrome is not so much a progesterone deficiency disease as a *progesterone response disease.* Just administering progesterone to a woman with premenstrual syndrome will not alleviate her symptoms unless progesterone receptors are available to transport the progesterone molecules to the nucleus of the target cells. Studying the characteristics of progesterone receptors enables us to understand why premenstrual syndrome is worse after a pregnancy or when menstruation has been halted, and why studies of twins and adopted daughters suggest that there is a genetic factor.

SPASMODIC DYSMENORRHEA

It has already been mentioned that spasmodic dysmenorrhea is the opposite of premenstrual syndrome, and there are several factors that suggest that an estrogen deficiency is the cause. For instance:

1) It does not start with the first menstruation, but only when ovulation occurs

2) It is relieved by a full-term pregnancy

3) If a pregnancy does not intervene, a gradual reduction in pain after the age of 25 is usual

4) The pain is relieved by the pill or by administering estrogen

5) The sufferers tend to be immature, with poor breast development and sparse hair in their armpits

6) It is frequently accompanied by acne.

In puberty, estrogen is responsible for the development of the secondary sex characteristics. In addition to pubertal breast development and the development and enlargement of the womb, it is especially responsible for developing the muscles of the womb and ensuring it has a good blood supply. Another important action of estrogen is the reduction of prostaglandin released by the endometrial cells lining the womb. Prostaglandins are chemicals released by cells when they are damaged. Many different types of prostaglandins have been found, and the particular prostaglandins released by endometrial cells are known as F-2-alpha. Research shows that the level of prostaglandin F-2-alpha in the blood is higher in women with spasmodic dysmenorrhea. If ovular menstruation occurs before there has been adequate estrogen to develop the muscle layer of the womb and control the secretion of prostaglandin F-2-alpha, the door of the womb, or cervix, will not be supple enough to open easily to allow the flow of menstrual blood. It is rather like trying to blow up a balloon the first time: it is hard to inflate, but once it has been fully inflated, the next time is easier. If the womb is gradually stretched during the nine months of pregnancy, then subsequently the door will open up at menstruation without pain. Or, if the muscles of the womb are gradually extended by the prolonged action of estrogen, the painful periods are gradually eased when the woman is in her mid-twenties.

Two Hormonal Types

Thus, it would seem that the two common menstrual problems, premenstrual syndrome and spasmodic dysmenorrhea, are related to problems of the two menstrual hormones—progesterone

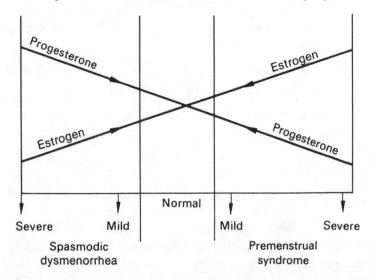

Figure 28 Arbitrary levels of progesterone and estrogen

and estrogen, respectively. Figure 28 is a diagram of the effect of these two hormone levels on an individual. A marked progesterone receptor deficiency will cause severe premenstrual syndrome. A moderately low estrogen level will only cause mild spasmodic dysmenorrhea, but a severe estrogen deficiency will cause severe period pains. Between these extremes lie those fortunate women who do not experience regular problems with menstruation. Although women may move up and down this scale slightly during their menstrual lives, they will tend to stay within the limits of the same group unless either progesterone or estrogen is given, or a pregnancy occurs. The two groups tend to have other common characteristics, which are discussed below.

PROGESTERONE-RESPONSIVE GROUP

Women with premenstrual syndrome tend to be fertile, but their pregnancies may be followed by postnatal depression, and they are more prone to depressive illnesses and high blood pressure during their life span. Of those who become pregnant, one in five is likely to have pre-eclamptic toxemia, with marked weight-gain and high blood pressure during pregnancy. Others blossom in pregnancy, being free from their usual premenstrual migraine, asthma, and depression, and will later look back on the last months of pregnancy as the healthiest days of their life. However, these women are more prone to develop postnatal depression. They will also tend to experience side effects if given estrogen, as they already have a high level of this hormone. Minor estrogen side effects include nausea, weight gain, headaches, and depression, but more serious ones, like thrombosis, are also possible. The pill contains estrogen and a synthetic progestogen and, as already mentioned, progestogens lower the normal progesterone level in the blood, making any existing premenstrual syndrome worse.

ESTROGEN-RESPONSIVE GROUP

Women with spasmodic dysmenorrhea grow out of their period pains, either following pregnancy or during their mid-twenties, and thereafter have trouble-free menstruations. These are the women who feel positively better on the pill, even preferring the ones with a relatively higher dose of estrogen, as these boost their low estrogen levels. At menopause, however, their already low estrogen levels are not helped by the declining estrogen output from the ovaries, and they are likely to develop menopausal symptoms early, even before menstruation has stopped. Unless they are given estrogen replacement treatment during the menopausal years, they are likely to be the ones who suffer most from the ending of menstruation.

As with other hormonal disorders, there is a strong family tendency, with daughters, sisters, and mothers belonging to the same menstrual hormonal group—either progesterone-responsive or estrogen-responsive. Studies in twins have shown that among identical twins, if one suffers from premenstrual syndrome then the other will too, whereas in non-identical twins, the incidence of premenstrual syndrome is the same as that found among sisters. Similarly, adopted daughters are likely to take their pattern from their natural mothers, not their adoptive mothers, with respect to having either premenstrual syndrome or spasmodic dysmenorrhea.

MISSED PERIODS

"Married hopes and unmarried fear
Are the common causes of amenorrhea"

Amenorrhea is the absence of periods, and the nurses' jingle quoted above is a reminder that the most common cause of missed menstruation is pregnancy. If the woman is single, it is more likely to be a delayed period. If she normally has a long cycle of 33–36 days, has not kept a record of her cycles, and has taken a chance during the month, then every day after the twenty-eighth day she is likely to fear that she might be pregnant. Unfortunately, the usual pregnancy tests cannot be used reliably until 2 weeks after the missed period, or 42 days since the last period, and this is a long time to wait. However, the usual early signs of pregnancy, such as morning sickness, getting up to urinate at night, and painful, enlarging breasts would be there. A new test called the HCG blood test can recognize a pregnancy within 7 days of conception, which is even before the missed period. HCG, or human chorionic gonadotrophin, is one of the special pregnancy hormones released immediately after conception. Serial ultrasound scans of the ovaries will also detect an early pregnancy within days of embedding in the womb. Both of these methods are expensive, however, and are not universally available. In an earlier hormonal pregnancy test, estrogen and progestogen tablets were given to a woman, and if she was not pregnant vaginal bleeding would occur within 48 hours. This test has now been banned worldwide because there is a risk of fetal abnormalities if the woman is pregnant.

It is quite normal for women to miss periods at puberty, during the first 3 years after menstruation begins, during breast-feeding, and again at menopause. Menstruation often starts to get shorter and the loss lighter around menopause before a period is actually missed.

Other causes of missed menstruation are found in the hormonal controlling system, for any upset to the hormonal pathway may disturb the menstrual rhythm. Stress is usually the most common cause:

> A friend, *Winifred*, visited us with her two children. When she returned home she found a fire engine outside and her house in flames. She stopped menstruating for 11 weeks.

Nor is it necessary for the stress to be unpleasant; missed periods can happen just as easily following happy circumstances:

> *Yvonne*, a 25-year-old graphic artist, had a wonderful romance on a Greek island. She stopped menstruating for 9 weeks after she returned.

In both these cases, the amenorrhea resulted from messages from the brain affecting the menstrual clock, situated in the hypothalamus.

Factors that disturb the other controlling centers in the hypothalamus (see Figure 21) will also upset the menstrual clock. A common example is rapid weight-change, brought on by anorexia nervosa or even strict dieting. Every woman has a critical weight level below which menstruation will stop, and it will not return until her weight reaches the critical level again. Women with a tendency to weight-loss and missed periods should weigh themselves at each menstruation, so as to learn their personal critical weight limits. Depressive illnesses may also delay menstruation, and again, the periods are unlikely to return until the depression passes. Other chronic systemic illnesses such as tuberculosis and acute rheumatic fever may also halt menstruation temporarily.

A lack of menstruation after stopping the pill may be caused by the ovaries being prevented from ovulating for so long that the menstrual clock has also stopped. This indicates that the menstrual clock does not restart automatically when the pill is discontinued. Often, however, there has been a weight-loss while the pill was being taken, and the weight-loss amenorrhea is revealed when the pill is stopped. When menstruation *does* restart after a long interval, the cycles are frequently found to be anovular. This means that although menstruation has restarted, ovulation has not and pregnancy is therefore impossible. Fortunately, this can be remedied by appropriate hormone treatment.

Too Much

Another problem is when menstruation goes on for too long, comes too often, or is too heavy—i.e., there is too much of it. Stress may be the cause, though not in those women who miss their menstruation at other times because of stress.

> *Zena*, the 45-year-old wife of a T.V. producer, bled for 9 weeks continuously, starting on the day her dream house was sold to a higher bidder without her knowledge.

There is an interesting story in Mark's Gospel:

> "And there was a woman who had a flow of blood for 12 years, and who had suffered much under many physicians, and had spent all that she had, and was no better, but

rather grew worse. She had heard the reports about Jesus, and came up behind him in the crowd and touched his garment. For she said, 'If I touch even his garments, I shall be made well.' And immediately the hemorrhage ceased, and she felt in her body that she was healed of her disease." (5, 25–29, RSV)

This incident can be interpreted in the light of our current medical knowledge about menstruation. The woman had great faith, and the tremendous emotional release of being able to go up and touch Jesus' clothes was sufficient stimulus to her menstrual clock to correct her prolonged menstruation.

Hormone therapy when taking the pill, especially the progestogen-only pill, may cause prolonged scanty bleeding, often referred to as "breakthrough" bleeding because it occurs between normal menstruations. This can be troublesome and is a sign that the treatment needs adjusting.

Occasionally, there may be bleeding at ovulation. This is usually lighter, and may last from 1 or 2 hours to 1 or 2 days. If there is no regular record, this bleeding may not be easily recognized for what it is. A menstrual chart will clearly show the difference between regular mid-cycle bleeding, which is harmless, and the totally irregular bleeding that needs gynecological investigation. However, one should always investigate bleeding at ovulation to ensure that it is not due to another cause.

Conditions that increase the surface area of the lining of the womb usually result in heavy or prolonged bleeding. Examples are polyps, or fibroids situated near the cavity of the womb. As there is always a chance that the extra bleeding may be the result of a malignant condition, it is always advisable to get a complete examination.

Sometimes, bleeding that is thought to be menstrual is caused by an ulcer, or erosion, at the cervix or opening of the womb. This can easily be detected by a doctor on examination, and cauterized.

18

After A Hysterectomy or Oophorectomy

Many women who have endured menstrual miseries each month for years dream of the day when those troublesome organs will be removed by one stroke of the surgeon's knife. Can anyone blame them? Already, hysterectomy is such a common procedure that it is known as the "Birthday Operation," to be celebrated in one's fortieth year, as this is the most common age for the operation. In the U.S.A. the phrase "total hysterectomy" is used to mean the removal of the womb, tubes, and ovaries, an operation known medically as "HBSO" or "hysterectomy with bilateral salpingo-oophorectomy." Medically, if the cervix is left after removal of the womb this is known as a "subtotal hysterectomy." Only if the whole womb including the cervix is removed do surgeons call it a "total hysterectomy." An oophorectomy is the removal of either one or both ovaries.

Today, the risks associated with the removal of the womb are minimal, but is it really the answer to a woman's prayers? It is no good asking the gynecologist, who sees the woman a few months later, examines the scar to see if it's well-healed, assures her that she'll never menstruate again, possibly prescribes some estrogen tablets, and says goodbye. It is better to ask the family doctor, who will care for this woman not just for one year, but for the next twenty.

There are many very good reasons for removing the womb and possibly the ovaries as well. At the top of the list comes the possibility of any malignancy. Sometimes it is done because of fibroids, when they are either so large that they interfere with another organ, or so numerous that they cause heavy menstruation resulting in anemia. Another good reason is because of endometriosis. There are also women who do it so as to be 100% contraceptively safe, who do not want to take the risk that goes with the pill or other methods of contraception, possibly because they have already tried these methods without success. A 42-year-old boutique owner told me that she had changed her gynecologist seven times before she found one who was prepared to remove her womb for contraception. She just did not feel convinced that sterilization would be reliable enough.

Far too many women have a hysterectomy in order to overcome their premenstrual syndrome. They would be better advised to have their condition treated with progesterone therapy. It is true that the symptoms are often so severe that drastic treatment is warranted; unfortunately, a hysterectomy is not the answer. One well-known gynecologist who diagnoses premenstrual syndrome explains to the woman that her trouble is caused by a progesterone deficiency. However, if she insists on a hysterectomy he operates, then refers her to the Premenstrual Syndrome Clinic for progesterone treatment.

The immediate post-operative weeks are usually pleasant and uneventful. However, whether it is only the womb or the womb and the ovaries that have been removed, there is now an irreparable break in the hormonal pathway (Figure 22), and the menstrual clock, which the surgeon did not touch in the operation, receives a severe shock. Within 6–8 days there is an increase in follicle stimulating hormone (FSH) from the pituitary, and within 8–10 days an increase in luteinising hormone (LH). The menstrual clock then reacts to the lack of information from the womb, and over the next 3 weeks there is a threefold increase in FSH and the amount of LH doubles and continues at the abnormally high level for years. This occurs whether the ovaries have been removed or not, although the increase is not as great if an estrogen implant is given at the time of operation.

The changes that accompany the surgical removal of the womb or ovaries are known as "artificial" menopause, and should not be confused with natural menopause. The changes in natural menopause occur gradually over several years, as the menstrual clock slowly closes down and the ovaries and womb shrink. In artificial menopause the changes are sudden and only affect the womb and/or the ovaries, leaving the menstrual clock intact, which continues its menstrual cycle until the time of natural menopause.

All goes well for about 6–12 months after the operation. Then the hormonal differences between the two groups of women discussed on pages 156–158 begin to show themselves. Those who previously suffered from premenstrual syndrome will find that their cyclical symptoms return. The husband may be the first to notice, and say something. Or the woman may recognize the telltale headache which previously ushered in a period, and which now assumes the proportions of a devastating migraine.

> Angela, the 48-year-old wife of a USAF colonel, had a successful hysterectomy for fibroids that had been causing heavy bleeding. She made an excellent recovery, until 9 months later when she suddenly had 4 days of extreme tiredness. She stayed in bed, blaming it on a virus. The following month it happened again; this time she stayed in bed for 6 days. Gradually, the duration of the tiredness increased until it took 2 weeks out of every month. It would start gradually, as a general tiredness, and she would manage to keep going for a few days, but soon bedrest became essential. The end of the attacks was quite definite, and afterward she was free of symptoms and could resume her normal social life.
>
> Her husband had kept a meticulous diary, from which a chart was made. She had already had 9 months of this distressing condition when I first saw her. Fortunately, it responded completely to progesterone treatment.

Premenstrual syndrome always increases in severity after a hysterectomy, and there may also be extra symptoms.

One woman, a part-time worker, was sent to me after she had been apprehended by the police for shoplifting. Two years previously she had had a hysterectomy, and prior to the operation she had suffered from premenstrual tension and headaches.

After the operation her premenstrual syndrome became worse, and for a few days of each month she would also experience breast fullness and feelings of unreality and confusion. She carefully charted these days on a calendar and related the episodes to the times of her expected premenstruum. She then arranged her work schedule to avoid stress on these inevitable confused days. In court she described the nature of the confusion, how sometimes she would come home having bought items she did not need, such as dog food when she had no dogs, highly spiced foods that she never ate, and underwear that was the wrong size. She would be in a daze and could not tell what was happening. The day of her offense had been such a day. Even when she was being taken to the police station by a plainclothes policeman after being charged, she thought the officer was a rapist who was driving her down an unknown road. The case was dismissed. She has since undergone progesterone treatment, and is now free from cyclical confusion and premenstrual syndrome.

In 1975, during a nationwide survey of the hormonal factors affecting migraines in women, researchers noted that women with a history of premenstrual syndrome said that the severity of their migraines had been increased by a hysterectomy. Their 3-month charts, giving the precise timing of migraine attacks, confirmed that the attacks were still occurring cyclically.

The need for women with cyclical symptoms to keep careful records and charts of their problems, even if they have had their womb or ovaries removed, cannot be emphasized too strongly. If it is difficult to record days of depression because the onset is gradual, it may be just as useful to record the days on which breast symptoms occur, as these are usually definite and commonplace. Alternatively, really good days may be recorded with a simple check mark [✓].

Brenda, 47 years old, began her consultation with a detailed account of how her husband had been moved from one town to another, and how she had made a suicide attempt within days of their move and had been hospitalized for several months. Within a week or two of her discharge, she moved back to her previous home, but made another suicide attempt the following week and was once again hospitalized. Only after giving a long and confused history, assisted by her husband, did she mention that she had had a hysterectomy and was now experiencing cyclical attacks of depression and moodiness. Once the cyclical nature of her symptoms was confirmed by a 2-month record, she was given progesterone treatment, which helped restore normalcy.

Two surveys done in 1975 indicate a high incidence of depression in women 1–3 years after a hysterectomy, with or without the removal of the ovaries. The depression appears to be greatest in those who were under 40 years at the time of the operation; those with a previous history of depression, especially postnatal depression; those in whom no gynecological abnormality could be found by the pathologist who examined the womb after operation (in one of the surveys, 45% of the wombs were reported to be normal); and those who had a history of marital problems.

Dr. Ronald Richards, a general practitioner in Oxford, England, observed that patients who had undergone hysterectomies often had medical notes bulging out of their files, so that one could tell at a glance that they had already been in and out of many hospital departments. His survey, confirmed by others, emphasized the high incidence of depression in those with a history of hysterectomy.

My paper on "The Aftermath of Hysterectomy," read at the Royal Society of Medicine in London in 1957, revealed that 44% of women had either been divorced, separated, or had seen a marriage counselor since the operation. One reason could be lack of understanding or empathy on the part of husbands who believe that the cause of the menstrual problems has been removed. One husband said, "She used to have a reason for it, but now she's quite unpredictable," and another, "I thought the operation would make her more even-tempered."

Another disturbing finding in the survey was that more than half the women gained more than 28 pounds in the year following their hysterectomy. How often is a woman warned *before* the operation that the odds are two to one that such a marked weight-gain will occur? The reason for the depression and weight-gain after hysterectomy may be related to the proximity of the menstrual clock to the mood controlling and weight controlling centers in the hypothalamus. (See Figure 21.)

There seem to be two types of post-hysterectomy depression: a cyclical depression and a continuous depression. The continuous depression is more likely to affect those who experienced spasmodic dysmenorrhea in their youth and have a tendency to be estrogen-deficient. These women respond very well to estrogen therapy, which needs to be continued through their depressive illness and well after the time of the natural menopause. The estrogen is given continually as there is no risk of it causing a build-up of the lining of the womb. If the depression is cyclical, it will respond to progesterone. This should also be given continually, even if ovulation is still occurring, as there is no longer the possibility of causing irregularity of menstruation.

If only a hysterectomy has been performed ovulation will continue, but with the interruption of the hormonal pathway there may be a gradual deterioration of ovarian function and a premature menopause. In these cases, as well as in the case of women who have had their ovaries removed, there is a decrease in bone mass and a risk of developing osteoporosis. These women need hormone replacement therapy; they will also benefit from moderate daily exercise and need to appreciate the importance of calcium in their diet.

A few women develop a high prolactin level, suggesting that the operation has caused a disturbance in the hypothalamic-pituitary mechanism. They usually respond well to bromocriptine, a drug that lowers the prolactin level.

In theory, the removal of the womb should have no effect on sexual activity. The vagina and clitoris are untouched and, if anything, sexual activity should be enhanced once the fear of becoming pregnant is permanently removed. In practice, however, some women who previously had a satisfactory sex life suddenly find that they have lost their sexual zest and enjoyment. If this happens it is worth seeking professional help; often testosterone can be a magic restorative.

Research has shown that when female apes have had their wombs removed, their partner rejects them. But if the ape is only given a mock operation, and the womb is not removed, the couple enjoy a natural sexual relationship. Whether a similar effect occurs in humans is not known because we do not carry out mock operations on humans.

19

Menopausal Miseries

It is only children who long to grow old—adults hate the very thought of it. This is especially true for women when menopause approaches. Many of them see this as a doorway leading to old age and senility—when it is really the gateway to an era of serenity, a time characterized by confidence, calmness, sophistication, stable moods, and endless energy.

Women are unique in the animal kingdom as the only females who outlive their reproductive function and can then enjoy up to half their lifespan without it. Their menstrual clock runs at its own individual rate, and the end of menstruation occurs according to an individual, pre-arranged plan. In some the clock runs on a little longer, in others it stops earlier.

The word "menopause" means the pausing of menstruation, and more precisely, the last menstruation. It is the reverse of menarche, but it cannot be timed as accurately because it is only seen in retrospect; only when there have been no menstruations for a year can it be dated exactly. Earlier, the term "climacteric" was used to cover the years before and after the last menstruation, a time when the changes were occurring in the reproductive system. Nowadays it is usual to use the term "menopause" more loosely to cover all the years of hormonal change.

HORMONAL CHANGES

As with all the changes Nature makes in our reproductive system, those at menopause are very gradual, taking between 5 and 7 years to complete. First, there is the occasional missed ovulation. Studies have shown that the occasional anovular cycles can occur up to 6 years before the last menstruation. Gradually, missed ovulations become more frequent, and the menstrual flow becomes lighter and more scanty. As the ovaries decline, the hypothalamus and pituitary try to stimulate them with an increased output of follicle stimulating hormone and luteinising hormone. But the ovaries are unable to respond; their production of estrogen and progesterone gradually decreases and over a few years stops entirely. (See Figure 29.) Thus the presence of menopause can be determined by blood tests showing a low level of estradiol and a raised level of FSH.

As mentioned earlier, the main functions of estrogen are rebuilding the lining of the womb after it has been shed at menstruation, altering the cervical mucus to assist fertilization, and breast development. It also has other functions that are especially important when the menstruating years are over. Estrogen promotes cholesterol balance, nourishes the circulatory system, increases the elasticity of the skin, and is involved in building up the bones. Throughout life, in both men and women, the adrenal glands build up progesterone from cholesterol and then convert it further into estrogen, testosterone, cortisone, and other steroids. When estrogen is no longer produced by the ovaries, it continues to be produced in the adrenal glands and in the peripheral tissues. After menopause it is this non-ovarian estrogen that has to fulfill the other functions for the blood, bones, and skin. Often, there is insufficient estrogen for these other tasks, either temporarily during the changeover time or permanently, and it is this lack of estrogen that is responsible for all the unpleasant symptoms of menopause. Then the woman, once her ovaries decline, is left to carry on without a sufficiency of this vital and powerful female hormone.

Up to the age of 40, narrowing of the arteries—particularly of the blood vessels of the heart—and coronary thrombosis is

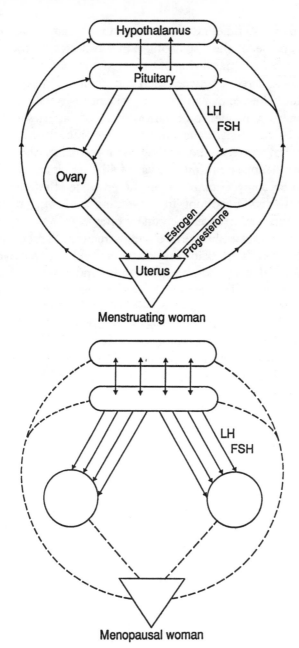

Figure 29 Hormonal pathways in menstruating and menopausal women

between 10 and 40 times more common in men than in women. After menopause, as the circulating estrogen decreases, there is a marked increase in narrowing of the arteries in women, so that gradually the difference between men and women decreases. But it is not until the age of 75 that the incidence is equal. After a hysterectomy the incidence of narrowing of the arteries and of the coronary vessels is increased four times as compared with premenopausal women. Also, among the few women who have a premature menopause before the age of 40, there is a sevenfold increase in coronary thrombosis. So the presence of estrogen in the blood is very important in preventing narrowing of the arteries and the occurrence of coronary disease.

Bones are not stable, unchanging structures. Throughout life, new bone cells are being laid down and old ones removed. This requires calcium, phosphorus, vitamins and other minerals, and also estrogen. This is why everyone, men, women, and children included, has a small amount of estrogen circulating in the blood. This estrogen is produced by the two adrenal glands. After menopause, women whose bodies have relied during their menstruating life on the estrogen produced by the ovaries may find they have insufficient estrogen being made by the adrenals. This leads to thinning of the bones. This loss of bone mass shows up on X rays, and 10 years after menopause it is present in 40% of all women. Although it can be controlled with estrogen therapy, it takes another 10 years before the X rays indicate any improvement.

Progesterone is no longer required to prepare the lining of the womb or the cervical mucus for possible pregnancy after menstruation ceases, but progesterone also has another function. All through life, in both sexes, progesterone is built up in the adrenal glands from cholesterol, and immediately converted into estrogen, testosterone, cortisone, and other adrenal hormones, or corticosteroids, which have various jobs to do throughout the body. As ovarian progesterone is only present in the blood stream for half of each cycle, the adrenals generally manage to make enough for their own needs during the menstruating years, and so they are usually capable of carrying on this task after menopause. This is why progesterone deficiency is no longer a problem after menopause, although if progesterone is given it can be converted into estrogen.

TWO HORMONAL GROUPS

Earlier, in Chapter 17, we discussed the two hormonal types, the estrogen-responsive and the progesterone-responsive. Most of our book has dealt with the progesterone-responsive group, and the problems that can be caused by premenstrual syndrome in the home, at work, and at play. At menopause we return again to the estrogen-responsive group, for these are the women whose menopausal sufferings begin earliest and are the most severe. This is illustrated in Figure 30, which shows that women who had spasmodic dysmenorrhea in their teens and then sufficient estrogen for normal menstruation nevertheless suffer most from menopausal symptoms. In fact, chances are that they will begin to experience menopausal symptoms while still menstruating regularly each month. They really need estrogen therapy at menopause, and probably for many years thereafter. Women who were in the normal category may require estrogen therapy during the changeover period, but will probably manage to

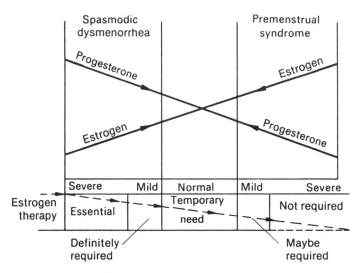

Figure 30 Need for estrogen therapy at menopause

make enough for their own requirements thereafter. Women who suffered from mild premenstrual syndrome may require estrogen temporarily when their menstruation first stops, but gradually they should manage without it. The severe premenstrual syndrome sufferers will probably have no need for estrogen, either during the menopausal years or later; they always have a high estrogen level, with ovarian estrogen supplemented by that produced in the adrenals.

In short, it is what we call in England a case of roundabouts and swings. Those who had greatest difficulties with premenstrual monthly problems can now look forward to a problem-free era, while those who had little trouble during their twenties and thirties will probably face the most problems at menopause.

Throughout the book I have avoided using the term "Hormone Replacement Treatment," or HRT, to avoid confusion. Both estrogen and progesterone are hormones, and both are used in replacement therapy. In the mind of the public and the media, HRT has become limited to the use of estrogen plus progesterone or estrogen plus progestogen therapy during menopause, while the letters ERT are used to denote estrogen replacement therapy. The term hormone replacement therapy has also been used for years by doctors when giving insulin to diabetics and thyroxin to those with hypothyroid disease.

AGE OF MENOPAUSE

In the United States the average age of menopause is 52 years, while in Britain it is 48 years, with a range of 45–55 years. Those whose menstruation ceases before they are 45 years old are said to have a "premature menopause."

The exact age of menopause is very individual. However, four factors can give some indication of whether it is likely to be early or late:

1) The age of menarche. Those who start menstruation early tend to finish late, so there is a "rainbow" effect, as shown in Figure 31

2) The hormonal group. Those in the estrogen-responsive

group have a tendency to finish menstruation early, while sufferers from premenstrual syndrome tend to finish after they are fifty

3) Genetic factors. If your mother, sisters, and aunts finished menstruation early, you may also expect to finish early. For this reason it is worth finding out at what age your mother had her last normal menstruation. If she had an easy change of life, the chances are that you, too, will have an easy time. If your mother suffered, make sure you receive the benefits of modern medicine

4) Smoking. A survey at a medical center in London showed that at 48–49 years, 36% of smokers were post-menopausal compared with 23% non-smokers; four years later, the figures were 89% for smokers and 71% for non-smokers. So smoking habits should also be considered when estimating the probable age at which menopause may occur.

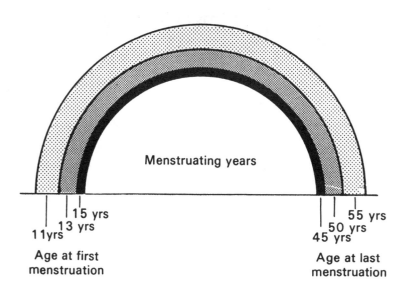

Figure 31 Relation between the age of menarche and menopause

PATTERNS OF ENDING

The charts of women who regularly record the dates of their menstruation show that the menstruating years end in a wide variety of ways. Three patterns are recognizable, but some women will find that their own individual ending covers more than one pattern:

1) There is a gradual ending. Where menstruation initially lasted 4 or 5 days, it gradually lasts 1 or 2 days, then only 1 day or even 1 hour monthly. Generally, the cycle is maintained and menstruation comes when expected

2) There is an occasional missed menstruation, possibly just one, and then menstruation resumes again for 2 or 3 months before another is missed. Gradually, there are more missed menstruations than actual menstruations, but each menstruation lasts the expected number of days, say 4–6 days

3) There is a sudden ending of menstruation, which had previously been regular, with the final menstruation lasting the normal or nearly normal number of days. This abrupt ending is most likely to coincide with a stressful event, such as a daughter's wedding, moving, or becoming a grandparent. This abrupt ending may even be the start of a depressive illness.

The effect of the first missed or delayed menstruation often depends upon the woman's recent sexual activity and desire for pregnancy. If she has not been sexually active, she may not notice the infrequency or absence of menstrual bleeding for a month or two. If she has been sexually active she may become concerned, and increasingly happy or unhappy with each additional day of missed menstruation. While the possibility of pregnancy is usually uppermost in the minds of women whose regular menstruation suddenly stops, after a woman is 45 she should always consider the possibility that menopause has begun. Comments by alarmed patients in this predicament include:

"I don't want to get my name in the *Guiness Book of Records* as the oldest mother in the world."

"I would hate to be drawing my old age pension when my child is at school."

And from a grandmother:

"My child would be younger than her niece."

It is usually quite easy for a doctor to tell if a patient is pregnant, or starting menopause. If she is pregnant her breasts will be full, she may have symptoms of morning sickness and of passing urine during the night, and on examination her vagina will be red and moist and the neck of the womb soft. If she is entering her menopause, her breasts will begin to decrease in size and firmness, she may experience menopausal symptoms, especially hot flashes, and on examination her vagina will be pale and dry and the neck of the womb firm and smaller.

HOT FLASHES

The most characteristic symptom of menopause is the "hot flush," or "flash." It is a sensation of burning heat, arising from the waist and passing up to the top of the head. It only lasts a few minutes, five at the most, and may either be visible, when the skin becomes flushed and beads of sweat appear, or invisible. Very few women indeed pass through their menopausal years without experiencing a single flash, which may range in frequency from only one or two a week to between 50 and 100 a day. Many women are embarrassed by them, but others working with women of their own age can laugh about them, believing that "a flash shared is a flash halved." Our grandparents used to say they were worth "a dollar a flash." They may be accompanied by palpitations, fluttering in the chest, or a feeling of choking, apprehension, or anxiety, and they are worse immediately after a hot drink or spicy food. If the hot flashes last longer than half an hour then there is likely to be some other cause for them.

The flashes can occur at night, when the woman may

awaken abruptly in a bath of sweat. These are known as "night sweats," and when the wife suddenly sits up and flings off the covers, the husband is more likely to be annoyed rather than sympathetic.

There is a story about a group of women undergraduates at Girton College, Cambridge, in the twenties, who were discussing the menopausal problems and hot flashes that their mothers and counselors were experiencing. They agreed that as they were all emancipated and fully understood the facts of life they would never have to suffer the same ordeals. They formed a Menopause Club, promising to keep in touch with each other and exchange full accounts of how they fared through that great age. When the time came, each one of them experienced the flashes and other menopausal symptoms to a greater or lesser degree, despite their full knowledge of the events of life. The flashes are thought to be caused by a sudden stimulus to the temperature controlling center in the hypothalamus, and are associated with a rise in FSH and LH from the pituitary, as well as a deficiency of estrogen. Thus they are hormonal and not psychological.

MENOPAUSAL SYMPTOMS

These symptoms are usually divided into two groups: specific symptoms, which are caused by estrogen deficiency and can be relieved by giving estrogen, and nonspecific psychological symptoms, some of which may be relieved by estrogen and some not, depending on the individual patient. These are illustrated in Figure 32. Nonspecific symptoms include tiredness, insomnia, irritability, depression, headaches, palpitations, anxiety, dizziness, forgetfulness, and absentmindedness. The psychological symptoms may be a secondary result of the primary symptoms, a so-called "domino effect." Thus the flashes, sweats, painful intercourse, and need to urinate frequently at night may cause insomnia and lead to tiredness, irritability, and depression.

Hot flashes and sweats are usually the first signs of estrogen deficiency. Lack of estrogen may cause the vagina to become dry, pale, thin, and less resilient. There is a change in the

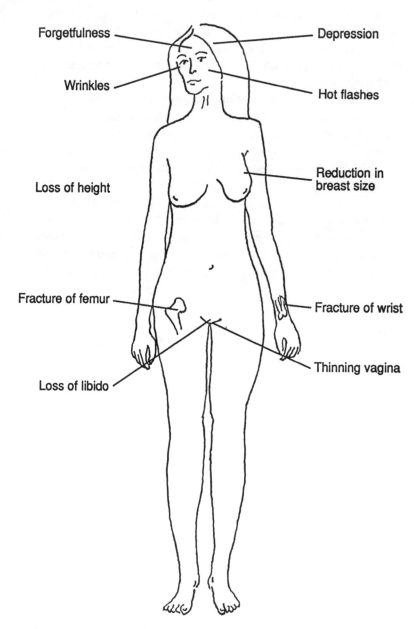

Figure 32 Signs of estrogen deficiency at menopause

acidity of the vagina, which leads to a change in the bacteria found there and a tendency to atrophic vaginitis and to infection. This in turn may cause itching, pain, or frequency in passing urine, especially at night (often misdiagnosed as cystitis). There is pain on initial penetration at intercourse and, ultimately, loss of sex drive.

The skin becomes paler and thinner and loses its elasticity, so that wrinkles develop, especially on the face around the eyes and mouth and on the neck. The soaring sales of cosmetics and beauty treatments and the demand for cosmetic surgery are evidence of the obvious distress caused by these symptoms of middle age.

The rheumatic-like pains that develop in the bones, muscles, and joints are due to the thinning of the bones. There is often considerable stiffness in the morning, and the pains tend to move around from one place to another over time. Sometimes the joints of the fingers become very painful and swollen, and as the pain and swelling decrease the joints may be left deformed and misaligned. These vague, generalized joint pains may be early signs of loss of bone mass, or osteoporosis, and are a warning that in the postmenopausal years, fractures of the wrist and the neck of the femur and crushed fractures of the spine are likely to occur. The typical "dowager's hump" at the top of the spine is also a sign of thinning of the bones, but this does not develop until the seventies.

Osteoporosis also causes a decrease in body height. Leonardo da Vinci, in his "Universal Man," showed that in humans the height equals the armspan. This is true for men and premenopausal women. As a woman's vertebrae become thinner after menopause, however, there is a decrease in height, with no corresponding decrease in armspan. If the difference between the armspan and height exceeds an inch and a half, it is an indication that the woman should receive long-term estrogen therapy. (See Figure 33.)

The greatest bone loss occurs early in menopause when menstruation is altering and becoming irregular, and for about 2 years after the last menstruation. Then the bone loss slowly reduces over the next 20 years. Gradually, the changes lead to

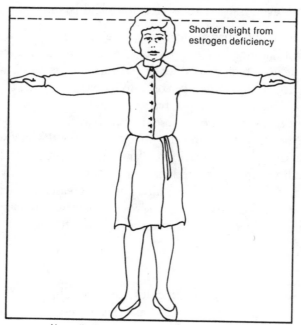

Normally the armspan equals the height, but if
estrogen deficiency occurs at the menopause
the armspan exceeds the height

Figure 33 Relation between armspan and height

the "little old lady" syndrome: "little" because height is lost, fat
is reduced, and possibly there is a dowager's hump; "old" because
this happens after menopause, and "lady" because the development of osteoporosis is about five times more common in
women than in men. All this results from the loss of estrogen,
for the estrogen receptors in the bones still require the hormone, but there is much that can be done to prevent it. (See
Chapter 21.)

The worst symptoms are the nonspecific ones, which can
lead to comments like:

"I think I must be going insane."

"I feel so harassed; the whole world seems to be resting on
my shoulders."

"It's even tougher than pregnancy and labor."

The mood changes at menopause are continual, not like premenstrual mood swings that last about 2 weeks and are then eased, at least temporarily. They can turn an easygoing woman into a nag, a high-strung person into a crying hysteric, a happy-go-lucky individual into a restless bundle of nerves, and an efficient housewife into an absentminded professor who puts the cat in the refrigerator and the milk out the door. Many women choose this time to leave the femininity rat-race, and their personality factors become more important—and possibly exaggerated. The woman's shape alters as her breasts begin to sag, and she develops middle-aged spread. There is a tendency for the thin to become even thinner and the fat to become obese.

DIAGNOSIS

Menopause is usually not difficult to diagnose clinically. The hot flashes are the most obvious characteristic, but it must not be forgotten that some antidepressants can also cause flashes. The thin skin, the graying hair, the wrinkles, the dry vagina, and deformed fingers and toes are all obvious signs. If further confirmation is needed, a blood test will show a rise in FSH, and if the bones are badly affected there will also be a rise in blood calcium and phosphates. A simple test that doctors perform is to examine some vaginal cells under a microscope. Cells with ample estrogen have a dark, well-marked nucleus. This is known as the Karyopicnotic Index (or K.I.) test, and is often done routinely when a cervical smear is performed. Its value is limited to the times when progesterone is absent, however, such as just after a period or long after the last period. If progesterone is present, the cells also lose their dark nuclei.

If the diagnosis is in doubt, the woman may be given a month's trial of estrogen. If she reports an improvement, the prescription can be repeated. While there is frequently a beneficial placebo effect from giving tablets, if the benefit is maintained over 2 or 3 months, it strongly suggests that it is the hormone treatment that is really beneficial.

The effect of menopause on sexual activity depends on a woman's experience during her menstruating years. If sex was important, then it is likely to be even more enjoyable once the fear of pregnancy is removed. If there never was much sexual excitement, then many think of menopause as a time when sexual activity may be slowed down or stopped. If estrogen is deficient, causing vaginal soreness and pain at penetration, the pain can be relieved by giving estrogen, either in the form of a cream applied locally or as tablets.

Some who talk and write—in error—about the "male menopause" describe it as a time when a man's sexual urge diminishes. This seems to be a kind of reverse chauvinism, which is doubly regrettable because it gives the impression that this is what is happening to women at menopause, which is quite wrong.

When Neuergarten was carrying out his study on attitudes toward menopause, he asked the loaded question, "What is the best thing about menopause?" Forty-four percent replied "not having to bother about menstruation," 30% said "not being worried about getting pregnant," and 14% said "a better relationship with my husband and greater enjoyment of sex life."

In 1969 the International Health Foundation studied the subject and interviewed 2,000 women who were between the ages of 45 and 55. Seventy-two percent agreed that after menopause it was good to be free from menstruation. Figures for the various countries ranged from 66% in Italy to 79% in the United Kingdom.

EMPTY NEST SYNDROME

Unfortunately, the menopausal years are often traumatic for women in other ways. It has been calculated that in the space of 5 years around her fiftieth birthday, the average woman will lose her mother through death, lose her daughter through marriage, and become a grandparent. There are also those homemakers whose children leave home for college or other employment, or who move because their husband makes a last career change or receives his final promotion. This has led psychologists to believe that all the miseries of menopause are just a woman's reaction to these losses—the so-called "Empty Nest Syndrome." While many women are upset by these events, and their turmoil may cause emotional impulses to reach the menstrual clock, in the majority of cases menopausal symptoms have a hormonal basis and respond well to estrogen therapy, which is fully described in Chapter 21.

20

❧

Helping Yourself

Once they know they have premenstrual syndrome, many women hope to find some way of coping with their monthly problems without having to see a doctor. Certainly, in mild cases it is important to try and help yourself, with the full knowledge that if you do not succeed, further help—and the most effective help—is available from any doctor who understands hormone therapy.

The desire to help herself was expressed by a nurse who wrote:

> "I always tended to be moody in my teens, but since my second pregnancy I have spells of hell, during which my doctor gives me tranquilizers. These help a little, but as a state-registered nurse, you can imagine that my training cries out, 'Treat the cause, not the result.' Please tell me what I can do to help myself."

And by another nurse, who pleaded:

> "There must be something more—I don't just want to take antidepressants forever when I feel so good and perfectly O.K. for half the month."

First let us deal with the "old wives' tales": there is no truth to the idea that you should not bathe, go swimming, or walk barefoot when menstruating or you will catch your death of cold. This idea probably began because, as we now know, pneumonia and viral disease commonly start during the premenstruum. It will not matter if you wash your hair when you are menstruating, although some women with very fine hair may find that a perm done at this time of the month will not stay in for long. Another false notion is that taking a cold shower will reduce the menstrual flow: the menstrual flow is going to come normally, in its own good time.

SPASMODIC DYSMENORRHEA

Proper relaxation and correct breathing is valuable for those with spasmodic dysmenorrhea. Unfortunately, the benefits are not so great for those with premenstrual syndrome. As mentioned earlier, the pain in severe spasmodic dysmenorrhea is similar to labor pains. In fact, the same nerves are involved in opening the entrance of the womb at childbirth as are needed at menstruation to let out the menstrual flow. Gradually, it is being recognized that the same relaxation exercises that women use in preparation for labor can also help to relieve the pain of dysmenorrhea. Some schools already teach older girls relaxation as part of their physical education, and dysmenorrhea sufferers have been helped by this. In Britain there is an organization called Relaxation for Living that exists purely to promote the teaching of relaxation, not just for that one day when a woman may be in labor, but to help both men and women to relax during their normal day to day living.

The National Childbirth Trust runs antenatal classes throughout Britain for those who are pregnant, and is helpful in providing the names of local teachers who are willing to help either an individual or a group of girls who have dysmenorrhea.

In the seventies, Drs. Margaret Chesney and Donald Tasto compared the effects of relaxation on college students in California. The students were initially separated into those with spasmodic dysmenorrhea and those with premenstrual syndrome; they were then divided by lottery into one of three treatment groups. One group received relaxation treatment at five weekly sessions and was told to practice the exercises daily at home. A second group attended a leaderless psychotherapy group for five weekly sessions, in which they compared their experiences of period pain. The last group was left untreated. All the students completed questionnaires regarding the severity of their pain before treatment and for three cycles after treatment was completed. Those who had spasmodic dysmenorrhea and took relaxation classes reported a dramatic improvement in their condition, which was sustained, but very few in the other groups benefited. So there does seem to be positive hope from simple treatment for those with spasmodic dysmenorrhea. However, if a woman is still crippled with pain after practicing the relaxation technique for a while, she should not hesitate to seek help from her doctor.

Prostaglandin inhibitors are considered safe enough today to be sold over the counter, and you may want to ask the advice of your pharmacist when choosing the best one for you. If your cycle is regular, start with half the normal dose for the 4 days before the pain is expected, and then increase to a full dose as soon as menstruation starts. An added advantage is that the total blood loss is usually reduced by about 25%.

It is a good idea to keep a menstrual chart at this time so that you know when to expect your next menstruation. You can also check if the pain comes every month, and if it has been improved by the simple self-help measures suggested above.

PREMENSTRUAL SYNDROME

Women who suffer from premenstrual syndrome will need different help. The *first* important thing is to keep a menstrual chart. You may use the type shown in Figure 3 or devise your own; it is the records that are important. If the chart shows the presence of symptoms during the paramenstruum, with freedom from symptoms during other phases of the cycle, you have PMS. Accept the diagnosis, but realize you are not alone: millions of other women are suffering like you. After an early television program on premenstrual syndrome many of the letters I received were from people who expressed this sense of relief:

"I went to sleep happy that night, knowing that I was not alone in my suffering."

"Just to know I wasn't mad .... I never dared talk about it; I thought I was the only one."

"All my problems were so peculiar I didn't expect anyone else to understand."

What is more, you may even want to try charting a friend's problems, such as colds, accidents, or temper tantrums. Some people have complaints month after month and never make the connection with menstruation, they just announce "Darn! I've got another cold."

Having accepted the diagnosis yourself, talk to others about it. Your husband, partner, or special friend should know and understand, and be told how to help you. If your PMS is severe, wait until you are feeling well, and then talk about it. Explain your feelings and fears, and how unhappy it makes you to periodically lose control. Share your deepest fears, maybe about harming your children, or attempting suicide. Discuss the problem that sometimes when you feel most down during the premenstruum, you nevertheless have an increased sex urge. Tell your partner that you still love him even when you're being awful and you can't help it and you want him to love you. Talk freely—there's nothing to be ashamed of. Tell the other people in your life so that they may understand you better. Discuss it with your family and friends so that they can appreciate your difficulties and stand by you. Explain it to your in-laws and to your employer—and don't forget that it is very important that men understand as well. Above all, see that your adolescent children understand it fully. If you are at school, you should discuss it with your teacher, or if you feel uncomfortable doing so, ask your mother or father to help.

One Sunday during a family dinner, my adolescent daughter broke a plate when she was clearing the dishes. "Don't worry, it's probably the wrong day of the month," commented my son. A few minutes later, my other daughter knocked over a glass and broke it. Trying to clear up the mess, I knocked a bowl of vegetables onto the floor. "I think we men better take care of the washing-up today," remarked my other son calmly. It seemed a far better way of dealing with a biological disturbance than getting annoyed with the two girls for their apparent clumsiness.

Mark in your diary when you expect your next period. Don't just assume that you have a cycle of 28 days; count the days of your last cycle and mark in the correct number of days for you. Consult your diary before arranging your next party, and avoid scheduling an interview, an examination, or a driving test on those awkward days. Arrange to have a perm or a tint during the postmenstrual week; it will take better then. If you are a journalist, be careful about what deadlines you accept. Teachers in high schools should set important homework 2 weeks ahead so that girls can do it when they are in their postmenstrual peak. If you have to take exams when you're feeling ill, write a note on your paper for the teacher.

At work, tell your employer or your personnel manager. It helps if they understand. If flextime is worked at your office, try to keep some hours or days in reserve to use when necessary. If there is shift work, try to get on the midday shift so that you have time to get up without hurrying and can dose yourself with progesterone if necessary before you start the day's work. PMS sufferers should avoid night shift work if at all possible, as nothing is more unsettling to the menstrual clock than mixing up night and day.

EATING HABITS AND DIET

In Chapter 16 the importance of the lower regulating mechanism for the control of blood sugar was discussed. This regulating mechanism is raised in sufferers of premenstrual syndrome, and it is therefore vital that they do not go for long intervals without some starchy food. The rule is to have small meals or snacks frequently, about every 3 hours. Instead of having two pieces of toast at breakfast, save one to enjoy with your midmorning coffee. At lunch, save half your sandwich (or whatever starchy food you usually have), so that you have something to eat in the afternoon. Save something from your evening meal to snack on before going to bed. It is really quite easy, and you will not need to eat more than your usual quantity.

Remember, whether or not you require progesterone therapy later, you will need to continue with the 3-hourly starchy diet. So even if you only *think* you have PMS, you should start on this diet while you are busy charting your symptoms.

Starchy food means anything made from flour, potatoes, rye, oats, and rice, and therefore will include bread, cookies, crackers, potato chips, and cereal. It does *not* include fruit, bananas, cheese, chocolate, and yogurt, which may be eaten with, but not instead of, starchy foods.

In Britain, the National Association of Premenstrual Syndrome (NAPS) promotes the 3-hourly starch rule and has a booklet of dietary advice. In 1989, members were asked if they had a "good," "moderate," or "poor" response to various treatments. Of the 250 replies, 68% reported a good response to the 3-hourly starch diet, with only 1% indicating a poor response. Of course such treatments are usually advocated only by non-profit charitable organizations, as there is no money to be made from them. It is a treatment that costs little, but does demand self-discipline. As one patient recently said, "I couldn't believe that the answer to all those miserable PMS days lay in the kitchen."

It is wise to carry emergency supplies of food with you always, ready for a long wait in line or a slow commute home. If your children are old enough, ask them to help you remember to eat every 3 hours. It's amazing how cooperative they can be. Make sure your partner understands too. Buy yourself a watch that beeps every 3 hours. Remember—it is essential to follow the 3-hour rule right through the cycle; it will not work if you limit it to the premenstruum. It should become routine—something that after a time you do naturally, without even thinking about it.

Recent work has shown that a "nibbling" or "grazing" diet lowers cholesterol and, in the overweight, helps weight-loss.

It is useful to fill in an attack form, shown in Figure 14, whenever you have a sudden attack of irritability, panic, or headaches. You will be surprised to see how often such problems start when no food has been taken for over 3 hours. If you transgress, and inadvertently go too long without food, don't be surprised to find that it may take you up to 7 days to feel well again.

If you follow the 3-hour rule faithfully, you may not need to limit your intake of liquids drastically, but do not exceed four cups a day. It is safe to eat a normal amount of salt, but not too much. Make sure, too, that your diet contains adequate protein and plenty of fruit and vegetables, and is a healthy and nutritious one.

If you drink alcohol, remember that half your usual amount will be enough to make you merry. Intoxication can occur easily during the paramenstruum in sufferers from premenstrual syndrome, so the other golden rules with regard to alcohol are important: don't mix grape and grain alcohol, or better still, don't mix your drinks; avoid drinking on an empty stomach; and don't drink and drive.

If constipation is a problem, or if you are unfortunate enough to have irritable bowel syndrome, then add a tablespoon of bran to your breakfast every day. This is not the same as bran flakes or bran cereal. It is natural bran, the stuff that looks and tastes like sawdust. It cannot be enjoyed alone, but can be added to other cereals, fruit juice, yogurt, or stewed fruit. Make it a daily habit, and after about 2 weeks you will appreciate its benefits with the regular, smooth opening of your bowels. In severe cases it may help to have 2 tablespoons of bran daily or have another helping of bran at night with cereals, soup, baked potatoes, stewed fruit, or yogurt.

There is no evidence that premenstrual syndrome is caused by a poor diet or a deficiency of any known vitamin or mineral. Problems caused by nutritional deficiencies can occur in men and women of all ages, and will be present throughout the month, although, as with all chronic diseases, the symptoms may be worse during the paramenstruum. Vitamins and mineral supplements are not needed in the treatment of premenstrual syndrome in women who follow a healthy diet. It is wise to avoid foods, particularly cereals, which are "vitamin enriched." This usually means vitamin B-6 has been added, and as explained on pages 212–214, an excess of vitamin B-6 can result in neurological symptoms. In general, self-medication with extra vitamins and minerals is ill-advised, can exacerbate problems or create new ones, and is a waste of money.

It is a good idea to give yourself extra rest during the second half of the cycle and, if possible, an afternoon nap. Even if you do not sleep, being in a relaxed state of semi-consciousness, lying in bed with the eyes closed is very helpful.

If a PMS sufferer has followed all this advice and is still miserable, she should see a doctor. Remember to take your chart with you, so that the doctor can confirm the diagnosis.

MENOPAUSE

Throughout this chapter simple self-help suggestions have been given for the treatment of menstrual problems. However, if menopausal symptoms are present, it is advisable to get medical advice sooner rather than later. Menopausal symptoms are due to estrogen deficiency, and if this is allowed to continue it can lead to osteoporosis. Your doctor is able to assess your personal risk factors, taking into account your family history, smoking habits, alcohol consumption, exercise, previous amenorrhea, and experience on the pill.

Avoid caffeine, hot drinks, and spicy foods as these are liable to spark off hot flashes. At night it may help to wear thin nighties, preferably cotton ones, to absorb the perspiration. If night sweats are a problem, then sheets and blankets are better than comforters, which keep the heat in much longer. It may help to have a starchy snack before going to bed, as sometimes night sweats are caused by low blood sugar sparking off an adrenalin spurt.

Your smoking habits and alcohol intake need consideration, as these can hasten osteoporosis. It is also important to get some daily exercise. This does not mean just normal walking to and fro as you putter about at home, but concentrated exercise for about 20 minutes, which leaves you breathless for at least 5 minutes. Choose what suits you best: a good brisk walk, a swim, a game of tennis, skipping, or using a bicycle machine in front of the TV while watching your favorite program. It must be daily exercise; once a week at the gym, club, or spa is not enough.

Think about your diet. Make sure you get sufficient calcium, which is found in milk, cheese, and fish, and that your daily intake of protein is adequate. Incidentally, white bread contains twice as much calcium as brown or wholemeal bread. Consider carefully if you need to lose weight; during these years of change, the fat tend to get fatter and the thin become thinner. If you are already below the ideal weight for your age and height, don't make matters worse by reducing your weight further, as fat cells increase the amount of available estrogen. Try to reach your ideal personal weight, taking into account your age and height.

If your nights are very disturbed, take an afternoon nap if you can. Sleep is important. Your skin will also benefit from some cream to combat the natural dryness that occurs now, and your greasy hair may need special shampoo.

If self-help proves inadequate for any of these monthly problems, further help is available from the medical profession. They have spent many years training, observing, and curing these problems and are helped by scientists, chemists, pharmacologists, biologists, and physiologists, who are all working to find a better understanding of the reproductive processes of women.

21

What Can the Doctor Do?

"How I resent those eight years of suffering now that I know how easy this is to cure."

"If only others knew that operations and being hospitalized are not the answer to these savage changes of mood . . . the real treatment is so simple."

The first steps a doctor will take when seeing a patient with menstrual problems is to confirm the diagnosis, check that there is no accompanying disease, such as unrelated depressive illness, and ensure that there is no evidence of malignancy.

"My doctor treats all of us with a D & C and that's it."

This comment may well be true, and is an indication of how careful the doctor is being in first eliminating the possibility of a precancerous condition in the body of the womb, which would not show up on a cervical smear or Pap smear. On the other hand, many gynecologists perform a dilatation and curettage at the drop of a hat, which does nothing to cure the hormonal imbalance.

Having confirmed the diagnosis, the doctor now has to decide whether to use hormone therapy, and if so, which one. Earlier chapters of this book have shown how deficiencies in the two menstrual hormones, estrogen and progesterone, result in completely different symptoms. Giving progesterone to a woman suffering from spasmodic dysmenorrhea or menopausal symptoms will only make her worse, and the same happens when estrogens are given for premenstrual syndrome. That is why a definitive diagnosis is essential before treatment can begin.

ESTROGEN THERAPY

The first estrogens used in therapy were non-steroids, and were quite different in composition from the natural estrogens found in the body. They included stilbestrol, dioenestrol, and hexoestradiol, that have since been shown to have some cancer-producing potential. They are never prescribed for oral use today, though dioenoestrol cream is sometimes recommended topically. It is the natural estrogens which are now prescribed, and their most important uses are in the treatment of spasmodic dysmenorrhea, to help mature the womb in adolescence, to substitute for failing ovarian estrogen at menopause, and in the contraceptive pill.

SPASMODIC DYSMENORRHEA

For many years estrogens were the standard treatment for spasmodic dysmenorrhea. However, current knowledge that women with this condition have high levels of prostaglandin F-2-alpha has revolutionized treatment. Today the drugs of choice are a whole range of prostaglandin inhibitors, which decrease the amount of prostaglandin in the tissues. These include ibuprofen (found in Advil, Motrin, and Nuprin), mefanamic acid (Ponstel), indomethacin (Indocin), and naproxen (Naprosyn). Some inhibitors are more specific against prostaglandin F-2-alpha, others are more effective in reducing the prostaglandin released when bone cells are damaged. Mefanamic acid is effective against prostaglandin F-2-alpha, and will both reduce dysmenorrhea and cut the menstrual flow by about 25%. The drug may be taken in a half-dose for the 4 days before the pain is expected, then increased to a full dose, 500mg three times daily, as soon as menstruation starts, and continued until the pain has ceased.

If estrogen is used, it is given in courses from day 5 for 21 days, and menstruation usually occurs within 2 days of stopping the hormone tablets. The first course will result in painless menstruation because it stops ovulation for that month. To remove spasmodic dysmenorrhea permanently, however, it is necessary to give many courses, perhaps for 6–12 months. During an investigation of period pains in the sixties, it was surprising how many girls wrote that they had received one course of estrogen, which had only helped in that one month and made no difference thereafter. It is a shame the girls were not told when they started the treatment that more than one course would be necessary to remove the pain altogether.

Estrogen can be given either alone or mixed with progestogens, as in the estrogen-progestogen pill. The advantage of the pill is that the person taking it can be sure menstruation will occur after 21 days. As the pills are prepared in carefully dated packs of 21, they are not easily forgotten; if forgotten, the mistake is easily visible and two tablets can be taken at once. The advantage of giving estrogen alone is that the amount of estrogen given can be varied, thus allowing for individual differences. However, bleeding does not always occur at the end of the course, and the person must be fully aware that estrogen used alone is not a contraceptive.

> *Dierdre*, 19, had been given estrogen in Australia to relieve spasmodic dysmenorrhea. She went to Britain on a 6-month holiday with sufficient tablets for her stay. After 4 months she realized she had missed her period and began to develop morning sickness. Her pregnancy test proved positive.
>
> As she had been taking a pill every day for 3 weeks and stopping for 1 week, just like all her friends who were on the pill, she assumed hers was also a contraceptive.

Parents often react unhappily if their daughters are given the pill to ease period pains. They need to understand that the girls are suffering, and the pill itself is not going to lead their precious daughters into promiscuity. The girls also need to be reassured that despite the terrible pains, their fertility is not in danger—in fact, the pain shows that they are ovulating and should not have much trouble conceiving.

Occasionally, women seeking treatment for spasmodic dysmenorrhea are also anxious to begin a family. In these cases a higher dose of estrogen may be given from day 5 to day 10 and day 18 to day 28 of each cycle, avoiding estrogen at the time of ovulation so that conception can occur.

When estrogen is used for spasmodic dysmenorrhea before the age of 25, side effects are rare because there is insufficient estrogen in the body and contraindications are hardly ever encountered.

ESTROGENS FOR MENOPAUSAL SYMPTOMS

When estrogens are given for menopausal symptoms the effect is dramatic. The number of daily hot flashes should decrease significantly within a week, and if the flashes still occur after 3 weeks, it is a sign that a higher dose should be used. In Britain, prescriptions for estrogens have increased by 50% over the last 4 years, suggesting that their value is now being fully appreciated.

Menopausal women who are still menstruating can have estrogen from day 5 until the time of their expected menstruation. For many women this means a 3-week course, while those with longer cycles will benefit from a longer course of estrogens. Otherwise they may go up to 2 weeks without treatment and risk the return of all their symptoms.

There is a concern that estrogen therapy may build up the lining of the womb so much in women who are not menstruating that it might predispose them to cancer. No one really knows whether this is so, but there is a solution to this problem that is worth considering. The shedding of the lining can be induced by progestogen tablets, which are taken for a few days and then stopped. Bleeding usually occurs within a day or two of stopping. The progestogen can either be added to the estrogen tablet and taken daily for 3 weeks and then stopped for a week, during which bleeding will occur, or it may be added only for the last 7–10 days of the 3-week course of estrogen. Some women may find that the added progestogens cause premenstrual syndrome; they will benefit from the addition of natural progesterone, which can be used rectally or vaginally, rather than the artificial progestogens, which are alien to the human body. Oral tablets of micronized natural progesterone are also available, and as only a small amount is required to provoke bleeding from an estrogen-primed endometrium, oral progesterone may be used.

Women, whether of menopausal age or younger, who have had their womb removed will also benefit from estrogen therapy. They do not need to have the progestogen added as there is no risk of them developing cancer of the womb.

Estrogen can also be given through an implant, in which one or more small pellets of pure estrogen are inserted, under local anesthesia, into the fat of the abdominal wall through a small incision in the skin. An implant relieves the patient of trying to remember to take daily tablets, but if any side effects develop it is not possible to remove the implant. It is particularly useful in women with menopausal symptoms who have had a hysterectomy, as after a hysterectomy it is not necessary to induce regular shedding of the lining of the womb. An estrogen implant can also be performed for younger women who undergo a hysterectomy in order to reduce the shock to their menstrual hormonal pathway. If there is any loss of libido, a pellet of testosterone implanted at the same time as the estrogen pellet will help.

Estrogen can also be absorbed through the skin, and plasters are now available that may be applied to the lower abdomen and changed twice weekly. The advantage of the plasters is that the estrogen does not pass through the liver but goes directly to the tissues requiring estrogen, and so the side effects are reduced. If the womb has not been removed it is still necessary for the woman to have regular vaginal bleeding, and this is arranged by giving the usual course of progestogen tablets.

The estrogen replacement therapy should be continued until there are no symptoms when the estrogen is stopped. If the woman is having a 3-week course of estrogen and has slight flashes during the week without treatment, she is not yet ready to stop. If she remains free of symptoms, then she can go for 10 days before starting the next course, and if that goes well, 14 days before starting the next one. If she can go 3 weeks without estrogen with no ill-effects, that is a sign that her body has learned to make the estrogen necessary for healthy bone metabolism, and she can discontinue hormone replacement. Just how long it may be necessary to continue treatment varies with each individual woman, and there are an unlucky few who may need to continue for 10 years or more.

The immediate side effects of estrogen are nausea, bloatedness, headaches, and depression. These will generally only occur in women who do not have an estrogen deficiency, such as women with premenstrual syndrome. The side effects ease when estrogen is stopped.

The question of whether or not there is any risk in prolonged estrogen therapy is hotly debated within the medical profession. There does not appear to be any risk with short-term treatments of less than 5 years. Follow-up studies of women who have had estrogen for 15 years or more are difficult to do, and yield confusing results.

When studying the incidence of cancer over the last 20 years one finds very unreliable data on whether the patients who developed cancer had ever taken any estrogen, what type it was, for how long and in what dosage it was taken, whether it was taken alone or with progesterone or progestogens, and also whether the patients were already at risk because of a positive family history of cancer of the breast or womb. Although the record-keeping is more precise now, one cannot expect a definitive answer for several years yet.

Anti-Estrogen Cancer Trials

In Britain a 10-year breast cancer study involving 30,000 women is currently being carried out. It is designed to test whether the established anti-estrogen drug tamoxifen, which is used to treat breast cancer, might also protect women who are predisposed to the disease. It is estimated that if tamoxifen produces a 30%

improvement in the incidence of breast cancer after it is taken for 5 years, the results will be detectable in 10 years, while a 50% improvement will be detected in 6 years.

On the other hand, long-term estrogen therapy has its benefits. The incidence in women of ischemic heart disease and strokes rise abruptly after menopause or after a hysterectomy or oophorectomy. It is likely that estrogen therapy reduces this risk, although again this cannot be positively proven for a few years yet.

For their own safety and peace of mind, women receiving estrogen therapy should see their physician at least every 6 months for a check on their blood pressure and weight, and for a breast exam, a general examination, and a cervical smear.

At a meeting of a women's group some years ago where I gave a talk on menopause, one member of the audience was very eager to tell the audience that her doctor had refused to give her estrogen for her hot flashes. Later in the talk, I listed the contraindications for estrogen therapy. These include a history of coronary thrombosis; angina; pulmonary embolism; deep vein thrombosis; cancer of the breast, womb or ovary; diabetes; liver disease; and high blood pressure. The same woman then rose and apologized, explaining that she was under treatment for high blood pressure. Today, however, high blood pressure is no longer regarded as a contraindication, although it would first need to be brought under control with hypotensive medication. It is better in this case to give estrogen plasters rather than tablets, to bypass the liver. In cases where estrogen is definitely contraindicated, relief of symptoms and prevention of osteoporosis may be achieved by progesterone therapy, which lowers blood pressure. Progesterone is normally made in the adrenals and converted into estrogen for use.

Some doctors feel that by eliminating the menstrual cycle they can also eliminate premenstrual syndrome. They advocate an estrogen implant to abolish menstruation, and then the addition of progestogens at the beginning of each month to ensure that there is a regular shedding of the lining of the womb. Unfortunately, it is not as easy as that. The menstrual cycle of women who undergo such treatment is disturbed for up to one year, and symptoms occur throughout the cycle so that their symptom-free postmenstruum is also forfeited. As we have already noted, cyclical symptoms will continue to occur after a hysterectomy or oophorectomy.

TREATMENT FOR
PREMENSTRUAL SYNDROME

A woman journalist conducted a small private survey to find out what different doctors were doing about menstrual problems. She noted the following as pretty standard answers.

"It (progesterone) doesn't work, and anyway, everybody's on the pill."

"It can only be given by injection."

"There's no proof it works."

"Placebo effects."

"Women are supposed to get some kind of masochistic pleasure from their pains."

These comments are typical of the attitudes that are delaying for many premenstrual syndrome sufferers the medical treatment and relief that is their right. The first answer is typical of the confusion in many doctors' minds between progesterone and progestogens. Progestogens do not work on premenstrual syndrome; progesterone does. (See pages 208–210.) The confusion is reinforced by the second part of the statement: "everybody's on the pill." The next comment is from those who may know the difference but are unaware of the progress that has been made in supplying progesterone in suppositories and pessaries. The third remark is symptomatic of our scientific age, which cannot accept the evidence of its own eyes without the support of strictly controlled clinical trials. "The proof of the pudding lies in the eating," or so people say. Hundreds of women, whose quotes appear throughout this book, needed no further proof of the value of progesterone in treating premenstrual syndrome than their own satisfactory experience. The other two remarks need no comment—they are like old wives' tales.

In fairness to doctors, it must be said that not many who are practicing today were taught anything about these hormones or hormone receptors when they were at medical school. There are increasing numbers of doctors who do know how and when to use estrogen and progesterone to alleviate the monthly sufferings of women.

PROGESTERONE

The first person to use the word "progesterone" was William Allen, who, with George Corner, first isolated this active constituent of the corpus luteum in the ovary. He proposed the name in December 1934, and 8 months later the principal scientists involved in work on this new female sex hormone accepted it. In 1943 Russell Marker emerged from the jungles of Central America and showed biochemists how to manufacture this pregnancy hormone—progesterone—from the roots of yams. However, once the biochemists had learned how to do this, the importance of progesterone itself was overshadowed by the many other steroids that could be obtained from it just by a subtle alteration of its chemical formula. In their laboratories biochemists converted progesterone into the lifesaving hormone cortisone, and it was also converted into progestogens, which are the basis of oral contraceptives and are used by countless women the world over. Progesterone is also converted into estrogens for use in hormone replacement therapy, and into testosterone for the restoration of male potency.

PROGESTERONE THERAPY

For many doctors progesterone is a forgotten hormone as far as treatment is concerned. Many doctors who use estrogen and know its possibilities and limitations are shy of using progesterone. One problem is that progesterone taken orally is not effective in the treatment of premenstrual syndrome, so it has to be given in other ways. These include suppositories that can be inserted into the rectum or vagina, injections, or implants. In

India work on monkeys suggested that progesterone could be absorbed into the blood stream when given nasally, so aerosols and nasal sprays were tried, but with little success. Later it was shown that progesterone cream applied to the noses of female rats was well-absorbed. An American pharmaceutical company, Nastech, reported in 1985 that tests done with women in North Carolina and in Yorkshire, England, used progesterone nasal cream with satisfactory results. There were hopes that this method of administration might revolutionize future progesterone therapy. However, there are no signs yet that Nastech are preparing to start the necessary trials of progesterone for premenstrual syndrome.

Whenever progesterone therapy is given, the patient must also follow the 3-hourly starchy food diet discussed on pages 189–191. It is rather like a diabetic on insulin: although the insulin is the lifesaver, the patient still needs to follow a strict diabetic diet.

When a woman with premenstrual syndrome who has been treated with progesterone returns to the doctor, it is often difficult to recognize her as the same person. The same woman who so often took an overdose of barbiturates during the late premenstruum, when everything was too much, will talk animatedly of the interesting evening classes she is now attending. The alcoholic who used to get into trouble each month will discuss the dream holiday she is planning. There is the husband who comes in to tell you about his wife, who is "now like the woman I married." There is the mother who is so delighted because "even the children are behaving better nowadays," the student who has happily passed her examinations, the epileptic mother whose children have been returned home to her care, and the asthmatic who drove to the Tower Bridge to ceremoniously throw all her aerosol inhalers into the Thames. For these women, who have suffered some of the serious consequences of premenstrual syndrome that we have discussed in earlier chapters, it is really no hardship to have to take their progesterone by pessary, suppository, or injection, instead of orally.

PROGESTERONE SUPPOSITORIES

Progesterone suppositories are small pellets of inert wax containing progesterone that are inserted into the vagina or rectum. The wax melts at body temperature releasing the progesterone, which is absorbed through the lining of the vagina or rectum and conveyed in the blood to where it is needed. The wax is expelled from the body, either moistening the vagina or mixed with the feces. Women who have vaginal infections are invariably treated with suppositories, and there are rarely any complaints. Suppositories are easy to insert into the anus, and were used by the ancient Egyptians, Greeks, and Romans for the administration of drugs to the rectum, where they are easily absorbed into the bloodstream. They have, however, never been a popular method of treatment in Anglo-Saxon countries and America.

During a recent vacation in Spain we were enjoying a pleasant evening with our Spanish hosts when their 4-year-old daughter emerged into the lounge complaining that she could not sleep because of an earache. The mother searched in her purse and gave the little one a suppository, probably a painkiller, which she took away and apparently used herself quite satisfactorily.

Many years of research preceded the introduction of commercially produced progesterone suppositories. The base in which the progesterone was dissolved had to be carefully selected, as the earlier ones tended to cause irritation and diarrhea. The temperature had to be carefully regulated while preparing the suppositories to prevent the formation of crystals, which produced painful pricking sensations when inserted. If the melting point of the suppository was too high, women with low body temperatures complained of grittiness.

Women who have learned to appreciate the value of progesterone no longer object to using suppositories. In practice, rectal and vaginal suppositories are interchangeable; it is usually left to the individual to choose what she prefers, and she may use both, on alternate occasions. Patients may generally use an extra suppository when an unexpected need arises, such as when there is a sudden surge of irritability, or a migraine threatens. Up to six 400mg suppositories can safely be used in a day; after all, during pregnancy the blood level of progesterone is so high that it would take 30 suppositories daily to reach the same level. If two suppositories are used simultaneously in the same orifice, the molten wax prevents further absorption of progesterone, so it is impossible for an individual to overdose with suppositories. Women should not insert a tampon at the same time as a suppository, because the tampon absorbs the progesterone and the woman receives no benefit.

The best time to give progesterone is determined by studying each individual patient's chart. In the normal case, it is given as suppositories from ovulation until the onset of menstruation. However, if symptoms continue until the second or third day of menstruation, then the progesterone should be continued until the fourth day. If symptoms start at ovulation, the progesterone should be started a couple of days beforehand. In short, the progesterone needs to be started at ovulation, or if later, at least 4 days before the symptoms are expected, and continued until menstruation has started. It is quite useless to give suppositories on alternate days from day 19 to day 25, which is how it was done in the double-blind controlled test reported by S. L. Smith (1975), which is often cited as proof that progesterone is ineffective because it was unsuccessful in that particular trial. The effectiveness of progesterone could not be demonstrated because it was used too late, without regard for individual variation in the length of cycle, for too short a time, and with too long an interval between each dose.

There is considerable variation in the absorption of progesterone by individuals: some absorb it quickly and others more slowly, some show immediate increases in the blood progesterone level, in others the rise or fall is slower. Furthermore, there is a small proportion of women, between 5% and 10%, who do not absorb progesterone effectively from the rectum or vagina, and need to receive it by injection. The absorption of suppositories is usually quick, and within 20 minutes there may be a rise in the level of progesterone in the blood, but the progesterone level may drop quite quickly too, and the effect is always over within 24 hours. In some women the effect only lasts 4 hours, which means that some women may need to take between two and six suppositories daily.

PROGESTERONE INJECTIONS

Progesterone injections last longer than suppositories. In some women they only need to be repeated on alternate days, while others need them daily. The absorption is more reliable, and so they are always used in critical situations, such as when a marriage is at a breaking point, or children are in danger of being taken away. Another advantage is that if they are given daily by a nurse, she can silently supervise those who need watching in the premenstruum—for instance, where there is a risk of suicide, child abuse, or excessive drinking. Injections are more convenient for patients in hospitals and are also used when suppositories have failed.

After a while, most patients learn the art of giving their own injections. Failing this, the husband or friend may be ready to learn the technique. Between the muscle fibers in the buttocks there are clumps of fat cells that form a cushion for us to sit on. The progesterone injection should be inserted into the buttock muscles, where it is absorbed by the fat cells and then gradually released into the blood. The injection can be given anywhere in the buttocks where there is a one-inch pinch of flesh, which means it cannot be given in the upper inner quadrant where the skin is closely attached to the end of the spine. The injections should not be given in the thigh or arm, where there are no fat cells between the muscle fibers.

PROGESTERONE IMPLANTS

Progesterone can also be administered by implants to those who have already had complete relief of symptoms with either suppositories or injections. The implant lasts for an average of 3–4 months, and occasionally for as long as 18 months. It is particularly useful for women who have had their womb removed, as they will not be troubled by the erratic menstruation that sometimes follows. It is also used for those who are forgetful in giving themselves progesterone, such as amnesiac alcoholics or drug users. One patient of mine who lived in Italy calculated that the cost of an annual implant plus the air fare from Rome was cheaper than the cost of daily suppositories.

However, a progesterone implant is not as convenient as an estrogen implant. More progesterone pellets are used, and they sometimes have a tendency to be extruded or pushed out. These incidents of extrusion are likely to occur at times of greatest progesterone need, such as during the premenstruum. The site of the implant may become inflamed, but this can be eased by giving progesterone injections for 5 consecutive days, thus temporarily giving the body an alternative supply.

A progesterone implant should not be given to those hoping to conceive within 12 months; those who may become anxious when their normal menstruation is replaced by an irregular, scanty loss or is possibly missed for up to 6 months; or those who must avoid premenstrual symptoms at all costs, such as the epileptic woman who may not realize that her implanted supply of progesterone is running low and has an epileptic attack at a most unfortunate or potentially dangerous time; and those whose normal daily requirement of progesterone is very high.

If progesterone is given daily by pessaries, suppositories, or injections and then stopped for some reason, menstruation will occur. This is similar to what happens when the level of progesterone drops and menstruation occurs in a normal cycle.

It is impossible to give an overdose of progesterone to a woman who has borne children. During pregnancy women are exposed to a thirtyfold increase in their blood progesterone level for 9 full months instead of a mere 2 weeks, and the body has learned to deal with that. On the other hand, in childless and immature women an excess of progesterone may very occasionally cause euphoria, restless energy, insomnia, and dysmenorrhea or uterine cramps similar to those suffered in spasmodic dysmenorrhea.

There are no contraindications for the use of progesterone. Also, there are no risks of progesterone causing cancer—in fact, progesterone is used in the treatment of some cancers, especially those produced in the vaginas of teenage girls who were exposed to stilbestrol (DES) during their fetal life, and advanced or recurrent cancer of the womb. If there is any possibility of candida (yeast infections) being present, this should be cleared up before pessaries are used, as progesterone may encourage candida to grow. It is also necessary to treat the partner with antifungal tablets to ensure that he does not reinfect the patient.

In Britain progesterone suppositories have been commercially available for 20 years and, in my personal experience, several thousand women have used them satisfactorily for many years. Suppositories in doses of 200mg and 400mg are distributed and marketed by Hoechst UK Ltd. under the trade name of "Cyclogest." In the United States for many years the Food and Drug Administration has permitted the commercial production of progesterone injections and also of 50mg progesterone suppositories for infertility patients with a luteal phase deficiency of progesterone. Tests are now proceeding for the use of higher doses. Meanwhile, it is quite legal for any pharmacist to make up progesterone suppositories of any strength on a doctor's prescription for a specific patient.

PROGESTOGENS

Because progesterone cannot be given orally, biochemists tried to make a synthetic preparation that could. They tried small alterations in the chemical formula, hoping to find a compound with slightly different properties; after all, progesterone, estrogen, testosterone, and cortisone all have very similar formulas, although they have quite different properties. Eventually they developed the progestogens, which are the basis of all contraceptive pills and gave rise to a multibillion dollar industry. When the progestogens were first discovered they were believed to be true progesterone substitutes. But, in fact, they had some properties of estrogen, some of progesterone, and some of testosterone. For example, if progestogens have been given during a pregnancy and the child is a girl, she is likely to show masculinizing effects in her genitals and be a tomboy, with marked aggression. This is quite different from the effect of natural progesterone, which is produced in such large quantities during pregnancy. Indeed, surveys have suggested that if progesterone is given to mothers before the sixteenth week of pregnancy for 8 weeks or longer, the child of that pregnancy has a tendency toward enhanced intelligence, with a good academic record, higher grades, and a better chance of reaching university level than control children whose mothers were not given progesterone.

There are many differences between progesterone and the various progestogens, but unfortunately there are still some doctors who do not realize this. Progesterone lowers the blood pressure, while progestogens raise it, and while progesterone raises the SHBG level, progestogens lower it. Progestogens are not accepted by progesterone receptors. Progesterone can relieve

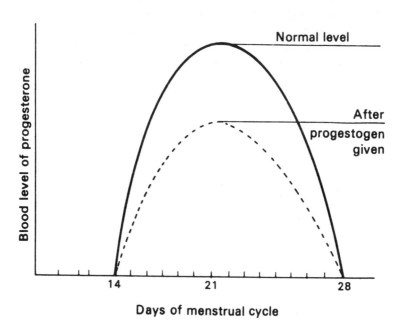

Figure 34 Effect of progestogen on the blood level of progesterone

water and sodium retention whereas some progestogens used in the pill, such as nor-ethisterone, cause retention of water and sodium. Progesterone is converted by the adrenals into all the various corticosteroids, which is not possible with progestogens. One function of progesterone is to maintain a pregnancy, but the progestogens cannot be used for this purpose. Some progestogens have an estrogenic effect as well, which is useful in the contraceptive field. The disposal of progestogens from the body differs from that of natural progesterone, which is excreted in the urine and feces as pregnanediol.

Progestogens also cause a lowering of the blood level of progesterone (see Figure 34), and this explains why women with premenstrual syndrome so often have difficulty in tolerating the pill, whether the estrogen-progestogen pill or the progestogen-only pill, and also other estrogen-progestogen preparations for menopause.

Some doctors believe that by eliminating ovulation and menstruation with the use of strong progestogens such as danazol, it is possible to eliminate premenstrual syndrome. Unfortunately, as mentioned earlier, this does not happen—it merely prolongs the premenstrual symptoms throughout the cycle. On the other hand, danazol is often the drug of choice in the treatment of endometriosis.

CONTRACEPTION

For those who have or have had spasmodic dysmenorrhea, the estrogen-progestogen pill is usually the best method of contraception. These women have a low estrogen level and benefit from the extra estrogen. In fact, many of them were unhappy when the high estrogen pills were removed from the market, because they felt so much better on a high dose. On the other hand, premenstrual syndrome sufferers tend to have difficulty with this pill, which causes an increase in headaches, weight-gain, depression, and nausea; they are also candidates for the more serious blood-clotting problems caused by the estrogen which can result in deep vein thrombosis or cerebral thrombosis. Furthermore, the progestogens tend to lower the normal progesterone level, making their premenstrual syndrome worse.

Women who are receiving progesterone treatment for premenstrual syndrome can take a progestogen-only pill from day 1 until day 11 and then start the normal progesterone dose until menstruation. Or they can start with a small amount of progesterone, say a 50mg progesterone suppository, from day 8, and take that until they start their normal course of progesterone, and continue it up to the start of menstruation. In this way they are contraceptively safe. Progesterone is nature's own contraceptive; it is present after ovulation and converts the thin vaginal mucus into a thick, sticky type that prevents sperm from entering the womb.

Sterilization is also not the ultimate and universal answer to the problem of contraception that it was once thought to be. Women with premenstrual syndrome may find the operation increases their symptoms (see page 33). Recently, Dr. B. W. McGuiness, a family physician in Cheshire, England, in a controlled series of tests, found that women who have bilateral tubal ligation suffered significantly more menstrual cycle disturbances post-operatively. His findings have since been confirmed by others.

CONCEPTION

Women on progesterone treatment who wish to conceive should start their progesterone 48 hours after their temperature chart shows ovulation has occurred. If they do not know when ovulation occurs, they should start on day 16 for cycles up to 28 days, and on day 18 for longer cycles. They should continue the progesterone until the pregnancy is confirmed, and then only stop if they are free from symptoms.

TESTOSTERONE

Testosterone, the male hormone, has occasionally been used in the past for the treatment of premenstrual syndrome, especially in those who have sore breasts premenstrually. It is effective, especially in giving energy, lightening or stopping menstruation, and easing the engorged breasts. However, it can have masculinizing effects such as hoarseness, deepening of the voice, and hair growth on the beard area of the face. Testosterone is also valuable in rapidly stopping menopausal flashes and depression when it is given in a combined tablet with estrogen. It also improves the sex urge and activity, and may be used in implants together with estrogen.

BROMOCRIPTINE

Bromocriptine is a drug that is capable of lowering a raised prolactin level. As explained in Chapter 16, sometimes a raised prolactin level interferes with the progesterone feedback pathway from the womb to the hypothalamus. There are reports from the Netherlands that patients with infertility and premenstrual syndrome have been successfully treated with bromocriptine. However, strictly controlled tests carried out on patients in England by Ghose and Coppen, using a different dosage, did not confirm these findings. Patients who appear to benefit from bromocriptine are those with marked water retention, painful and engorged breasts throughout the cycle, those who have lost their sex interest, those who have recently had postnatal depression, and women with raised prolactin levels.

PYRIDOXINE

Pyridoxine, or Vitamin B-6, has been recommended for women who become depressed when using estrogen-progestogen contraception, and for menopausal women receiving estrogen replacement therapy. Unfortunately, worldwide clinical tests have failed to show the value of pyridoxine in women with well-diagnosed premenstrual syndrome. The recommended daily requirement of B-6 is only 2–4mg, yet doses of ten or even 100 times that amount are often prescribed. Schaumberg, an American neurologist, had the task of giving animals peripheral neuritis so that a possible curative drug might be developed. Peripheral neuritis is a painful, chronic, debilitating disease occurring commonly in diabetics and alcoholics. The animals were given

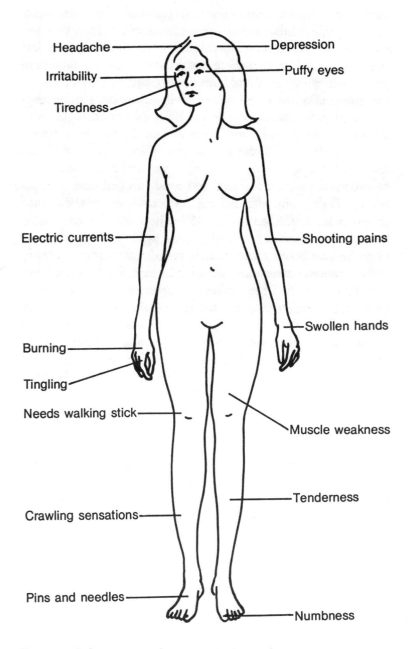

Figure 35 Symptoms of vitamin B-6 overdose

vitamin B-6 (pyridoxine), and the team of which he was a member reported that pyridoxine overdose could cause degeneration of the peripheral sensory neurons (nerve endings) in dogs and rats. In 1983 Schaumberg and his colleagues reported peripheral neuropathy resulting from massive pyridoxine overdose in five women and two men, who had degeneration of their peripheral sensory neurons revealed at biopsy. In my practice, with my son, Dr. Michael Dalton, we tested all the women currently taking pyridoxine. Of the 172 women whose blood pyridoxine level was above the normal range, we noted that 60% had neurological symptoms of pins and needles, numbness, oversensitivity of the skin with itching and crawling sensations, and muscle weakness. (See Figure 35.) There was no correlation between the incidence of neurological symptoms and the dose of pyridoxine being taken, which varied from 25mg to 500mg daily. However, there was a correlation with the length of time that pyridoxine had been taken. Irrespective of whether it was taken daily or intermittently, the neurological symptoms tended to appear after 6 months, regardless of the dose. Nor did it matter whether pyridoxine was taken alone, with other B vitamins, with other vitamins, or with magnesium—the incidence of neurological symptoms of overdose was the same. Fortunately, when pyridoxine is abruptly stopped there are no withdrawal symptoms, no further progression, and a gradual recovery from the temporary disabilities.

CLONIDINE

Clonidine, marketed under the name of Dixarit, is a drug used for lowering blood pressure. In very small doses it may be used to relieve menopausal flashes in those who, for some reason, are unable to tolerate estrogens. It only acts on the flashes, however, and is of no value in relieving other estrogen-deficiency menopausal symptoms, such as vagina and skin thinning, joint pains, and psychological symptoms. One menopausal lady who always had a beautifully coiffured head of white hair refused to have a further course of estrogens, which, although they cured her menopausal flashes and depression, caused some of her white hair to become gray again. She opted for Clonidine, at least for a few months, until the psychological symptoms began to get her down.

Diuretics

It is best to avoid diuretics. Any help they give to those with water retention is temporary, and it is too easy to repeat them indefinitely, always taking more and more until the balance of sodium and potassium is disturbed. Diuretics do not help premenstrual tension, depression, or irritability; they only relieve the symptoms caused by water retention, such as bloatedness, weight-gain, and swollen ankles. Once one is addicted to diuretics, it is difficult to stop taking them. It has to be done gradually, first reducing from four to three, then three to two, at monthly intervals, and always in the postmenstruum. When the dose is down to one daily, continue the reduction, taking the diuretic on alternate days, then every third day and every fourth day, until it is finally stopped.

Potassium

A lowered blood potassium level may occur in those who have been taking diuretics for a long time, those who have food cravings and prolonged dieting, and those who complain of exhaustion and muscle weakness throughout the cycle. These women should have their blood potassium tested, and if a low level is found, they should take potassium tablets and change to a potassium-sparing diuretic until the deficiency is corrected.

22

A Fairer Future

This book is written with the aim of spreading the news that the once-a-month miseries of countless women can be, and are being, successfully treated and relieved. It is also written to help men understand and appreciate the menstrual problems of women, and become partners in helping them through their difficult days. That you are reading this book brings hope that the aim will be achieved.

Menstrual problems are widespread and often incapacitating. Their effects are felt by all classes, all ages, and both sexes. Currently it is possible to eliminate dysmenorrhea, premenstrual syndrome, and menopausal problems by giving hormone therapy, but although treatment is possible, it is not yet universal. Menopausal clinics are now well-established, so that gynecological help is available nationwide for the relief of symptoms related to the change of life. The recognition of premenstrual syndrome is not as widespread, although there have been many encouraging developments since the first edition of this book.

In 1983 Mrs. Lindsay Burton Leckie and Mrs. Pat Cannon, both of whom suffered from premenstrual syndrome and had benefited from progesterone therapy, founded the National PMS Society, a nonprofit, all-volunteer, educational and support network consisting of 91 affiliated groups throughout the United States. Their goals were to educate the medical and lay community in the identification and treatment of premenstrual syndrome, to promote an awareness of the existence of premenstrual syndrome among the general public, and to assist women by offering emotional support and updated information. Though the Society is now defunct, much of its good work is being carried on by independent groups, which offer literature and newsletters on premenstrual syndrome. Other activities include walk-in counseling, telephone hotlines, public meetings, workshops and seminars, and fund-raising for premenstrual syndrome research. For a list of clinics and support and information groups, see the Appendix on page 235.

A SPECIALTY OF
THE FAMILY PHYSICIAN

Premenstrual syndrome should really be a specialty of family practice, and should be mastered by every family physician. Someday, every generalist and consultant will be able to diagnose, treat, and manage all cases of premenstrual syndrome which come within his or her orbit. The long-term follow-up of a chronic disease such as premenstrual syndrome is best done by the physician of continuing care, rather than in hospitals, with their ever-changing junior staff and their need to discharge patients as soon as possible to make way for new ones. At present, however, this goal is a long way off.

Gynecologists tend to be satisfied with a clear physical examination. They may reassure themselves with a D & C, then refer the patient back to the family doctor. Endocrinologists feel they have more serious diseases to occupy their time and rarely trouble themselves with disturbances of the menstrual hormones, especially at a time when there are not enough useful hormonal estimations to confirm a diagnosis and determine the dosage of hormones needed. Psychiatrists do occasionally recognize the syndrome, and prescribe antidepressants or tranquilizers, but they may next see the patient during her symptom-free postmenstruum and decide she no longer needs care. Neurologists will investigate all cases of epilepsy and migraines to ensure that no lesion is present, and discharge the patient. The chest physician treats the asthma, the rhinologist treats the allergic rhinitis, the orthopedic surgeon and rheumatologist treat the backache and painful joints, the dermatologists treat the herpes and neurodermatitis, and so on. But even if all the menstrually related symptoms are known to these specialists, the overall diagnosis may easily be ignored.

One dream has come true. The University of Oklahoma is leading the world in having a department of Premenstrual Syndrome, with a multidisciplinary staff working together to bring relief to sufferers of premenstrual syndrome. Their responsibility includes conducting clinics for the diagnosis and treatment of premenstrual syndrome, teaching medical students and residents, and organizing research aimed at helping women worldwide. Hopefully, by the time the next edition of this book is needed, other universities in other countries will appreciate the need and follow this shining example.

WHY IS PMS SO BADLY TREATED?

Having read so far in the book, you may be wondering: "If progesterone and estrogen are such successful treatments, why aren't more doctors using them?" And, "Why do some doctors prefer to use a less successful drug that only brings partial relief to a few patients with mild symptoms, rather than one that brings complete relief to most patients with mild and severe symptoms?"

There is no simple answer to these perfectly reasonable questions. Some answers are contained in earlier chapters, and there are other reasons which come under three broad headings:

1) Doctors are essentially conservative

2) Commercial considerations play a large role

3) There is a lack of consultancy and treatment facilities for PMS.

Very few doctors practicing today have had any real training in diagnosing or treating what we know to be the world's most common disease, premenstrual syndrome. Doctors are themselves wholly responsible for the diagnosis and treatment of their patients. They have the right and the responsibility to protect their patients and themselves, so they are naturally reluctant to use treatments which are new, or are not yet fully established as safe and effective. However, they are also responsible for increasing their knowledge of the subject for, on the average, a general practitioner in Britain will have about 50 women in his or her practice needing treatment for premenstrual syndrome. Another factor is that doctors receive little training in nutrition, and rarely if ever ask a patient for a detailed account of her usual or previous day's diet. Some may say that there is no time to take a dietary history, but this could easily be done by a nurse or assistant.

One cannot ignore commercial pressures in today's world. Progesterone is not protected by a patent, so no drug manufacturer will benefit financially from marketing it. The costs of clinical trials and of gathering the necessary evidence to convince the F. D.A. of the effectiveness of progesterone in the treatment of premenstrual syndrome are high, and if any manufacturer succeeds in getting a license there is no guarantee of profit, because any other manufacturer could produce a similar product. Vitamins and minerals, on the other hand, are a good source of profit because they can be advertised to the general public and sold over the counter without a medical prescription and without the need to prove their effectiveness. However, they offer no special benefit to women with premenstrual syndrome.

General practitioners who have patients with a condition that is hard to diagnose can send them to a specialist. But to whom can they send their cases of premenstrual asthma or premenstrual sinusitis, which has been confirmed by a menstrual chart? Not to a gynecologist or endocrinologist or psychiatrist. Consulting specialists in the field of premenstrual syndrome just don't exist.

These are partial answers to our two questions, and they reflect a situation that is changing rapidly. The number of doctors who can diagnose and treat menstrual problems increases all the time. If more clinics could be established and training courses instituted, the number of undiagnosed and untreated sufferers would steadily decrease.

HOPE FOR THE FUTURE

In 1986 the Dalton Society, an international medical society of doctors, was founded with the object of furthering knowledge of and research into premenstrual syndrome. The Society has held conferences in Los Angeles, Chicago, Tulsa, and Oklahoma City, attended by doctors worldwide, where research papers have been read and discussions held on improvements in treatment and a better understanding of the causes of premenstrual syndrome. The research papers read at the 1989 conference are published in *Steroids*, a refereed medical journal. There are also "friends of the society" who, although not in the medical field, contribute funds and their energy to the alleviation of the problems brought on by premenstrual syndrome, surely a worthwhile charity deserving of generous support.

PREMENSTRUAL SYNDROME CLINICS

In Britain in 1985 the National Commission for Women passed a resolution calling the government's attention to the need for greater undergraduate and postgraduate education on premenstrual syndrome, and the need for training teachers, social workers, police, and lawyers about this subject.

If premenstrual syndrome clinics are to be established, the general practitioner will need to take the lead, assisted by a psychiatrist and gynecologist. Only the general practitioner deals with the whole range of PMS symptoms, and has an idea of the effect on the family. Before GPs can fulfill this role, however, they need specialized courses in diagnosing and treating menstrual problems. Medical students should also be made more familiar with the subject during their undergraduate training. General practitioners need to learn the art of adjusting menstruation for important events, knowing the methods and the risks, how to help women best utilize their peak postmenstrual days, and how to recognize those women with dysmenorrhea and premenstrual syndrome who need urgent treatment.

The need for greater public education and awareness is obvious. And a very real opportunity exists for the media to educate a public that welcomes human interest stories and news of medical possibilities. We must remember, however, that doctors do not like to be told by the press what treatment they should give their patients. Education on these subjects is already included in the curriculum of British high schools. Hopefully, this will help both the women and men of tomorrow to have a greater understanding of the problems, and the solutions which are available.

Menstrual problems are estimated to cost American industry 8% of the total wages paid. Surely it would be better to invest a fraction of that amount in menstrual clinics and training schemes for doctors, in order to recover all that lost time.

School and university examinations can be made more fair by adjusting schedules to the needs of women, and by offering alternative dates where possible, especially for laboratories and oral examinations.

A better understanding of the relationship between premenstrual syndrome and social and domestic violence would enable premenstrual baby battering to be correctly diagnosed, understood, and treated. This could reduce the problems of children being separated from their parents and taken into foster-care, and criminal proceedings against the mother.

Confronted with all these issues, one might think it would be best to abolish menstruation altogether at those times when conception is not required. As discussed, this can be done by the prolonged administration of progestogens, but it is not yet completely safe. Initially, there tends to be occasional breakthrough bleeding, and then after a year or two, there is a subtle change in the woman's personality: she becomes harder and more efficient, with a loss of sex interest. Is the price worth it? There is also the technique of menstrual aspiration, which women can learn to do themselves, in which they suck the menstrual flow from the womb through a thin flexible plastic tube and complete menstruation in one minute or less. Unfortunately, menstrual hormones may be upset by this procedure and their smooth ebb and flow disturbed. Many women eagerly hope that removal of the womb will solve the problem of menstruation, but as mentioned earlier, removal of the womb often upsets the hormonal pathway, and the end result may be worse than the condition before the operation.

In the last century, essayist John Ruskin reminded us that "the true wealth of the Nation was running to waste" because most children had no education. The same applies today in respect of the lack of education and understanding about premenstrual syndrome. Discussion of menstruation and menstrual problems should be as open and unrestricted as the discussion of sex, and information about menstruation should be available to all.

A quotation from Henry David Thoreau runs:

> "If you have built
> Castles in the air,
> Your work need
> Not be lost;
> There is where they
> Should be.
> Now put foundations under them."

Let us get down to work.

GLOSSARY

Abortion—death of the fetus

Adrenal glands—two glands situated above the kidneys and responsible for producing numerous hormones

Adrenalin—one of the hormones produced by the adrenal glands

Amenorrhea—absence of menstruation

Analgesic—drug taken to relieve pain

Anovular—without ovulation

Anorexia—loss of appetite

Antenatal—before childbirth

Antidepressant—drug to remove depression

Anus—exit from the alimentary canal, or back passage

Bromocriptine—drug which lowers the prolactin level

Candida—yeast infection

Cervical smear—test for the diagnosis of cancer of the neck of the womb

Cervix—neck of the womb

Climacteric—change of life

Corticosteroids—hormones produced in the cortex of the adrenal glands

Cystitis—inflammation of the urinary bladder

Diuretics—drugs capable of increasing the amount of urine passed

Dysmenorrhea—pain with periods

Dyspareunia—pain on intercourse

Embryo—developing ovum up to end of eighth week after conception

Endocrine gland—organ releasing hormones into the blood to act on distant cells

Endocrinologist—one who studies the effects of the endocrine glands

Endometrium—inner lining of the womb

Estrogen—hormone released by the ovary

Fallopian tubes—two tubes leading from the ovaries to the womb along which the egg cells pass

Fetus—developing human from 3 months to birth

Follicle stimulating hormone—hormone produced by the pituitary acting on the ovary to ripen the follicles and produce estrogen

Galactorrhea—fluid in the breast when not breastfeeding

Glaucoma—disease of the eye characterized by raised pressure in the eyeball

Glucose—a form of sugar found in the blood

Gonadotrophin—hormone produced by the pituitary acting on the gonads, either testes or ovary

Gynecology—study of the diseases of women

Hemorrhage—loss of blood, bleeding

Hormones—chemicals produced by the glands which have an action at a distant site

Hyperglycemia—raised blood sugar

Hypoglycemia—lowered blood sugar

Hypothalamus—specialized part of the brain concerned with control of body functions

Hysterectomy—surgical removal of the womb

Implant—pellets of drugs inserted into the tissues

Intermenstruum—part of the menstrual cycle not covered by the premenstruum or menstruation, usually days 5 to 24

Intrauterine device—small contraceptive appliance inserted into the womb

Labor—birth of baby

Lactation—breastfeeding

Lethargy—excessive tiredness

Libido—sex drive

Luteinizing hormone—hormone produced by the pituitary which causes ovulation and the production of progesterone

Menarche—first menstruation

Menopause—last menstruation marking the end of the child-bearing era

Menstrual clock—specialized portion of the hypothalamus responsible for the cyclical timing of menstruation

Menstrual cycle—time from the first day of menstruation until the first day of the next menstruation

Menstrual loss—bleeding at menstruation

Menstruation—monthly bleeding from the vagina in women of childbearing age

Metabolism—building up and breaking down of chemicals in the body

Migraine—severe form of headache

Mittelschmerz—abdominal pain accompanying ovulation

Ovary—reproductive organ containing egg cells

Ovulation—release of egg cell from the ovary

Ovum—egg cell

Paramenstruum—premenstruum and menstruation

Pituitary—gland situated at the base of the brain and controlling many other glands

Placebo—inactive or inert substance with no curative value

Placenta—organ which develops within the womb responsible for feeding the fetus and for the production of the hormones of pregnancy

Postmenstruum—the days immediately after menstruation

Postnatal—after childbirth

Potassium—mineral present in blood and cells of the body

Premenstruum—the days immediately prior to menstruation

Preovulatory—the days immediately before ovulation

Progesterone—hormone produced by the ovaries, adrenals, and by the placenta during pregnancy

Progestogen—man-made drug used for contraception, which was once thought to be a substitute for natural progesterone

Prolactin—hormone produced by the pituitary gland

Puerperium—time after childbirth

Pyridoxine—vitamin B-6

Sodium—mineral present in the blood and cells of the body

Spasmodic—coming in spasms

Sterilization—operation to permanently prevent conception

Synchrony—occurring at the same time

Syndrome—collection of symptoms which commonly occur together

Testosterone—male hormone

Therapy—treatment

Thrombosis—blood clot

Trauma—injury

Urethritis—inflammation of the urethra

Uterus—womb

Vagina—passage leading from the exterior of the body to the mouth of the womb

Vaginitis—inflammation of the vagina

Other Publications
by the Author

BOOKS

1964: *Premenstrual Syndrome*. William Heinemann Medical Books, London. (Translated into Spanish.)

1969: *The Menstrual Cycle*. Penguin Books, Harmondsworth, London; Pantheon Books, Random House, New York. (Translated into Spanish, Portuguese, French, Dutch, German, Swedish, Norwegian, and Danish.)

1977: *Premenstrual Syndrome and Progesterone Therapy*. William Heinemann Medical Books, London; Year Book Medical Publishers, Chicago.

1978: *Once A Month*. Fontana Paperbacks, London; Hunter House, California, U.S.A. (Translated into Dutch.)

1980: *Depression After Childbirth*. Oxford University Press, Oxford. (Translated into Dutch and Japanese.) Revised 2d edition, January 1989.

1984: *Premenstrual Syndrome and Progesterone Therapy*. William Heinemann Medical Books, London; Year Book Medical Publishers, Chicago. Revised 2d edition.

1987: *Once A Month*. Fontana Paperbacks, London; Hunter House, California, U.S.A. Revised 3d edition. (Translated into Japanese.)

1990: *Once A Month*. Hunter House, California, U.S.A. Revised 4th edition.

1990: *Premenstrual Syndrome Illustrated*. Peter Andrew Publishing, Worcestershire, U.K. (Spring 1990.)

1990: *Premenstrual Syndrome Goes to Court.* Peter Andrew Publishing Co., Worcestershire, U.K. (Mid-1990.)

ORIGINAL PAPERS

9 May 1953: "The premenstrual syndrome." *British Medical Journal,* vol.i, p.1007. Joint authorship with Raymond Greene.

6 November 1954: "The similarity of symptomatology of premenstrual syndrome and toxaemia of pregnancy and their response to progesterone." *British Medical Journal,* vol.ii, p.1071. BMA Prize.

May 1955: "Discussion on the premenstrual syndrome." *Proceedings of the Royal Society of Medicine,* vol.48, no.5, pp.337–347 (Section of General Practice pp.5–15).

December 1955: "Progesterone in toxaemia of pregnancy." *Medical World.*

June 1957: "The aftermath of hysterectomy and oophorectomy." *Proceedings of the Royal Society of Medicine,* vol.50, no.6, pp.415–418 (Section of General Practice, pp.13–16).

17 August 1957: "Toxaemia of pregnancy treated with progesterone during the symptomatic stage." *British Medical Journal,* vol.ii, pp.378–381.

17 January 1959: "Menstruation and acute psychiatric illnesses." *British Medical Journal,* vol.i, pp.148–149.

1959: "Menstrual disorders in general practice." *Journal of the College of General Practitioners,* vol.2, p.236.

12 December 1959: "Comparative trials of new oral progestogenic compounds in treatment of premenstrual syndrome." *British Medical Journal,* vol.ii, pp.1307–1309.

23 January 1960: "Early symptoms of pre-eclamptic toxaemia." *The Lancet,* pp.198–199.

30 January 1960: "Effect of menstruation on schoolgirls' weekly work." *British Medical Journal*, vol.i, pp.326–328.

12 November 1960: "Menstruation and accidents." *British Medical Journal*, vol.ii, pp.1425–1426.

3 December 1960: "Schoolgirls' behaviour and menstruation." *British Medical Journal*, vol.ii, pp.1647–1649.

30 December 1961: "Menstruation and crime." *British Medical Journal*, vol.ii, pp.1752–1753.

June 1962: "Controlled trials in the prophylactic value of progesterone in the treatment of pre-eclamptic toxaemia." *Journal of Obstetrics and Gynaecology of the British Commonwealth*, vol.LXIX, no.3, pp.463–468.

July 1963: "The present position of progestational steroids in the treatment of premenstrual syndrome." *Medical Women's Federation Journal*, pp.137–140.

1964: "Notes on the use of the menstrual chart." *Drug and Therapeutics Bulletin*.

October 1966: "The influence of mother's menstruation on her child." *Proceedings of the Royal Society of Medicine*, vol.59, no.10, pp.1014–1016, (Section of General Practice with Section on Paediatrics). BMA Prize.

October 1967: "Influence of menstruation on glaucoma." *British Journal Of Ophthalmology*, vol.51, no.10, pp.692–695. BMA Prize.

1968: "Ante-natal progesterone and intelligence." *British Journal of Psychiatry*, vol.114, pp.1377–1382.

December 1968: "Menstruation and examinations." *The Lancet*, pp.1386–1388.

4 April 1970: "Children's hospital admissions and mother's menstruation." *British Medical Journal*, vol.ii, pp.27–28.

March 1970: "The importance of menstrual dates." *Update* pp.310–314.

June 1971: "Prospective study into puerperal depression." *British Journal of Psychiatry*, vol.118, no.547, pp.689–692.

December 1971: "Puerperal and premenstrual depression." *Proceedings of the Royal Society of Medicine*, vol.64, no.12, pp.1249–1252, (Section of General Practice, pp. 43–4).

19 February 1972: "Ovulation symptoms and avoidance of conception." *The Lancet*, pp.437–438.

June 1973: "The general practitioner and research." *The Practitioner*, vol.210, pp.784–788.

January 1973: "Progesterone suppositories and pessaries in the treatment of menstrual migraine." *Headache*, vol.12, no.4, pp.151–159.

13 May 1974: "Premenstrual ankle edema in young girl." *Journal of American Medical Association*, vol.228.

1973: "Migraine in general practice." *Journal of the Royal College of General Practitioners*, vol.23, pp.97–106. Migraine Trust Prize Essay 1972.

April 1975: "Do it yourself." *British Migraine Association*, Migraine Newsletter.

August 1975: "The effect of progesterone on brain function." *Proceedings of the Acta Endocrin Congress*, Amsterdam.

1975: "Postpubertal effects of prenatal administration of progesterone." *Society for Research in Child Development*.

October 1973: "The influence of menstruation." *Update*, pp.883–839.

July 1975: "Premenstrual syndrome." *Update*, pp.121–128.

October 1975: "Food intake prior to a migraine attack—study of 2313 spontaneous attacks." *Headache*, vol. 15, no.3, pp.188–193.

January 1976: "Migraine and oral contraceptives." *Headache*, vol.15, no.4, pp.247–251.

1976: "Prenatal progesterone and educational attainments." *British Journal of Psychiatry*, vol.129, pp.438–442. The Charles Oliver Hawthorne BMA Prize Essay 1976.

April 1976: "A clinician's view." *Royal Society of Health Journal.*

April 1976: "Menstruation and sport." Chapter in *Sports Medicine* 2d edition. J.P.R. Williams and P.N. Sperryn, Eds. Edward Arnold, London.

1976: "Treatment of the premenstrual syndrome." *Journal of Pharmacotherapy*, pp.51–55.

1976: "Bromocriptine and premenstrual syndrome." *Pharmacological and clinical aspects of Bromocriptine*. R.I. Bayliss, P. Turner and W.P. McClay, Eds. M.S.C. Consultants, London.

19 December 1977: "Premenstrual syndrome with psychiatric symptoms." *Journal of the American Medical Association*, vol.238, no.25, p.2729.

11 August 1978: "Synthetic progestins vs. natural generic progesterone: pharmacologic properties." *Journal of the American Medical Association*, vol.240, no.6.

12 August 1978: "Menarcheal age in the disabled." *British Medical Journal*, no.2, p.475. Joint authorship with Maureen E. Dalton.

1979: "Intelligence and prenatal progesterone: a reappraisal." *Journal of the Royal Society of Medicine*, vol. 72, pp.397–399.

November 1979: "Food intake before migraine attacks in children." *Journal of the Royal College of General Practitioners*, no.29, pp.662–665. Joint authorship with Maureen E. Dalton.

December 1979: "Intelligence and prenatal progesterone." *Journal of the Royal Society of Medicine*, vol. 72, p.951.

26 September 1980: "Cyclic posthysterectomy symptoms." *Journal of the American Medicine Association*, vol. 244, no.13, p.1497.

15 November 1980: "Cyclical criminal acts in premenstrual syndrome." *The Lancet*, pp.1070–1071.

1981: "The effect of progesterone and progestogens on the foetus." *Neuropharmacology*.

1981: "Violence and the premenstrual syndrome." *Journal of Police Surgeons*, Great Britain.

17 April 1982: "Legal implications of premenstrual syndrome." *World Medicine*.

1982: "Overview of premenstrual syndrome." Chapter in *Behavior and the Menstrual Cycle*. R. Friedman, Ed. Marcel Dekker, New York.

1982: "Premenstrual syndrome and its treatment." *International Medicine*, vol.2, no.2, pp.10–13.

1982: "What is this PMS?" *Journal of the Royal College of General Practice*, pp.717–719.

1983: "Premenstrual syndrome: a new criminal defense?" *California Western Law Review*, vol.18, no.2, pp.268–286. Joint authorship with Lawrence Taylor.

1984: "The depression of PMS and menstrual distress." *Mimms*, March 1984, pp.32–3.

1984: "Menstruation and migraine." *Migraine Matters*, vol.2, no.1, pp.6–8.

1984: "Diagnosis and clinical features of premenstrual syndrome." Chapter in *Premenstrual Syndrome and Dysmenorrhoea*. M. Y. Dawood, Ed. Urban and Schwarzburg.

18 May 1985: "Pyridoxine overdose in premenstrual syndrome." *The Lancet*, p.1168.

June 1985: "Progesterone prophylaxis used successfully in postnatal depression." *The Practitioner*, vol. 229, p.507.

September 1985: "Erythema multiforme associated with menstruation." *Journal of the Royal Society of Medicine*, vol. 78, p.787.

1985: "Menstrual stress." *Stress Medicine*, vol.1, pp.127–133.

March 1986: "Vitamins: a new perspective." *Mimms Magazine*.

1986: "Premenstrual syndrome." *Hamline Law Review*, vol.9, no.1, pp.143–154.

1986: "Should premenstrual syndrome be a legal defence." Chapter in *Premenstrual Syndrome: Ethical implications in a Bio-Behavioural Prospective*. B. F. Carter and B. E. Ginsburg, Eds.

January 1987: "Nasal absorption of progesterone in women." *British Journal of Obstetrics and Gynaecology*, vol. 94, pp.84–88. Joint authorship with M. E. Dalton, D. R. Bromham, C. L. Ambrose, and J. Osborne.

1987: "The efficacy of progesterone suppositories as a contraception in women with severe PMS." *British Journal of Family Planning*, vol.13, pp.87–89. Joint authorship with M. E. Dalton and K. Guthrie.

1987: "Premenstrual syndrome and thyroid." Accepted for publication by *Integrative Psychiatry*.

1987: "Characteristics of pyridoxine overdose neuropathy syndrome." *Acta Neurologica Scandinavica*, vol.76 pp.8–11. Joint authorship with M. J. T. Dalton. Awarded Cullen Prize.

1987: "What is this PMS?." Chapter in *The Psychology of Women—Ongoing Debates*. Mary Roth Walsh, Ed. Yale University Press.

1987: "Incidence of PMS in twins." *British Medical Journal*, vol.295, pp.1027–8. Joint authorship with M. E. Dalton and K. Guthrie.

June 1987: "Trial of progesterone vaginal suppositories in the treatment of premenstrual syndrome." Letter in *American Journal of Obstetrics and Gynecology*, vol.156, no.6, p.1555.

1987 Commentary on: "Premenstrual syndrome and thyroid dysfunction." *Integrative Psychiatry*, vol.5, pp. 179–193.

1988: "Treating the premenstrual syndrome." *British Medical Journal*, vol.297, p.490.

1988: "Progesterone for premenstrual exacerbations of asthma." *The Lancet*, 2; 8912 p.684.

September 1989: "Successful prophylactic progesterone for idiopathic postnatal depression." *International Journal of Prenatal & Perinatal Studies*.

1989: "Postpartum depression & bonding." *International Journal of Prenatal & Perinatal Studies*, pp.225–226.

May 1990: "Hypothesis: the aetiology of premenstrual syndrome is with the progesterone receptors." Accepted for publication in *Medical Hypothesis*.

1990: "Do progesterone receptors have a role in PMS." Accepted for publication in *International Journal of Prenatal & Perinatal Studies*.

APPENDIX

———— ❧ ————

PMS Clinics and Support Groups in the U.S.A.

This appendix is compiled from information received up to April 1990, and is arranged in two lists. The first list comprises clinics with a medical director who accepts that premenstrual syndrome is a hormonal disease. The second list includes the names of clinics, self-help groups, and other organizations with a non-medical director, whose approach to PMS may be psychological, nutritional, educational, or herbal. Some are lay organizations which act as local referral agencies, others organize self-help groups, and most are able to put premenstrual syndrome sufferers in touch with physicians who understand progesterone therapy. Both lists are organized alphabetically by state and by zip code within each state.

Those marked with a † have a member of the staff who has attended at least one lecture by Dr. Dalton. Those marked with an * have a member of the staff who has attended a 2–4 day training course with Dr. Dalton.

While every attempt has been made to make these lists useful, they cannot remain comprehensive or up-to-date.

These addresses and related information are only supplied
as a service to the reader seeking further information. The inclusion of any group does *not* constitute a recommendation or
endorsement of any kind by the author or the publisher. The
author and publisher cannot be held liable for any results from
self-treatment, or treatment at any of the facilities listed in this
book.

GROUPS WITH A MEDICAL DIRECTOR

Alaska

† The Health Care Center   (907) 562-7643
5001 Arctic Blvd., Ste. 100   W. Scott Kiester, D.O.
Anchorage, AK 99503   Jan Kiester, R.N.

Arizona

† 3330 Gynecology Ltd.   (602) 264-3267
3330 N. 2nd Street, Ste. 211   Donald E. Lee, M.D.
Phoenix, AZ 85012

Rene E. Allen, M.D.   (602) 886-5994
6632 E. Carondelet   Rene E. Allen, M.D.
Tucson, AZ 85710

California

† PMS Center   (213) 276-1151/1152
9201 Sunset Blvd., Ste. 906   Lloyd Byron Greig, M.D.
Los Angeles, CA 90069

Connie Chein, M.D.   (213) 274-8310
9242 Olympic Blvd.   Connie Chein, M.D.
Beverly Hills, CA 90212

Saint Mark Medical Group   (213) 587-1175
7648 Seville Avenue   Amal Y. Zaky, M.D.
Huntington Park, CA 90255   Emad M. Gharghoury

† PMS Treatment Clinic   (818) 447-0679
150 N. Santa Anita, Ste. 755   Holly Anderson, Director
Arcadia, CA 91006   Dino Clarizio, M.D.

† PMS Medical Clinic of So. Cal.   (818) 798-9431
2595 E. Washington Blvd., Ste. 105   Thomas L. Riley, M.D.
Pasadena, CA 91107   Rayne Dawson, P.A.-C.

San Diego PMS Clinic   (619) 297-3311
591 Camino de la Reina, Ste. 533   Lori A. Futterman. M.D.
San Diego, CA 92108   M. E. Ted Quigley, M.D.

PMS Treatment Center Of Riverside   (714) 784-1460
4000 14th Street, Ste. 504   William David Moore, M.D.
Riverside, CA 92501   Josefina Abdur-Rahman, R.N.P.

* PMS of Orange County   (714) 837-1510
24953 Paseo de Valencia, Ste. 7C   Frank Wm. Varese, M.D.
Laguna Hills, CA 92653

Women's Lifecare Medical Centers   (714) 974-3472
500 S. Anaheim Hills Road, Ste. 200   Harinder Grewal, M.D.
Anaheim Hills, CA 92807   Ria Gagnon

Burlingame PMS Clinic   (415) 697-7211
1828 El Camino Real, Ste. 504   William Rosenzweig, M.D.
Burlingame, CA 94010   Corinne Carrigan

* June A. Engle M.D., M.S.   (415) 866-9529
5201 N. Canyon Road, Ste. 310   June Engle, M.D.
San Ramon, CA 94583

Kathryn Morris, M.D.   (408) 458-1441
626 Frederick Street   Kathryn Morris, M.D.
Santa Cruz, CA 95062

North County Clinic   (707) 822-2481
785 18th Street   Gena C. Pennington, M.D.
Arcata, CA 95521

Colorado

PMS Treatment Center   (303) 869-1504
Women's Hospital at AMI St. Luke's   William E. Fuller, M.D.
601 E. 19th Avenue   Judith Ensign, M.S., R.N.
Denver, CO 80203

Florida

The Florida PMS Clinics, Inc.   (305) 271-8808
11400 N. Kendall Dr., Ste. 212   E. Gail Brown, M.D.
Miami, FL 33176   Vera Selmore, M.D.

Georgia

Bernard Mlaver Medical Clinic   (404) 448-4535
3700 Holcomb Bridge Road, Ste. 6   Bernard Mlaver, M.D.
Atlanta, GA 30092

PMS Institute Of Atlanta
5 Concourse Parkway   Edward M. Portman, M.D.
Atlanta, GA 30328   Glenda Gismondi

Illinois

* Fox Valley PMS Center   (708) 897-5616
648 N. Randall Road   William H. Woodruff, M.D., OB-GYN
Aurora, IL 60506   Peg Sechrest, R.N.C.
                             Judy Barr, C.S.T.

Iowa

Women's Health Center   (515) 424-1100
23 N. Federal Avenue   Laurie Summers, M.D.
Mason City, IA 50401   JoAnne Hunt, A.R.N.P.
                  Nancy Lindgren, M.S.W.

Kansas

† Glenn O. Bair, M.D.   (913) 267-3025/5689
2300 West 29th Street, Ste. 123   Glenn O. Bair, M.D.
Topeka, KS 66611   Charlotte Elder, R.N.

Michigan

William Beaumont Hospital   (313) 551-5000
Division of Reproductive Endocrinology   William Keye, M.D.
Department of Ob/Gyn
3601 13 Mile Road
Royal Oak, MI 48073

Minnesota

Wellness Center of Minnesota   (507) 345-7898
Good Counsel   William D. Manahan, M.D.
Mankato, MN 56001   Carl Lofy, S.T.D.
                     Linda Hachfeld, R.D.

Missouri

† PMS Center of St. Louis   (314) 727-3087
950 Francis Place, Ste. 114   John B. Bennett, M.D.
Clayton, MO 63105

† PMS Program Center   (314) 997-3333
941 Gardenview Office Parkway   Joseph G. Nouhan, M.D.
St. Louis, MO 63141   Patricia C. Coughlin, M.S.N.
                      Catherine L. Fox

† PMS Carecenter   (816) 276-7376
Rockhill Medical Building, Ste. 224   Mary C. Cortner, M.D.
6700 Troost Avenue   Joan Wood
Kansas City, MO 64131

Joe A. Gardner, M.D., Inc   (417) 782-2660
2700 McClelland, Ste. 303   Joe A. Gardner, M.D.
Joplin, MO 64804

Montana

Planned Parenthood of Billings   (406) 248-3636
PMS Program   Jean Omelchuck, M.A., L.P.C.
721 N. 29th St.   Clayton McCracken, M.D.
Billings, MT 59101

North Carolina

PMS Clinic   (919) 748-4479
Dept. of Family & Community Medicine
Bowman Gray School of Medicine   Elizabeth Philp, M.D.
300 S. Hawthorne Road   Marcia Szewczyk, M.D.
Winston-Salem, NC 27103

† Duke University Medical Center   (919) 684-5322
PMS Clinic   John Steege, M.D.
Box 3263   Anna L. Stout, Ph.D.
Durham, NC 27710   Sharon L. Rupp, R.N.C.

Ohio

PMS and Menopausal Treatment Center   (419) 422-6717
1816 Chapel Drive, Ste. I   M.C. Parekh, M.D.
Findlay, OH 45840

Oklahoma

* Ruth Miller, D.O.   (918) 299-1200
2931 E. 91st Street   Ruth Miller, D.O.
Tulsa, OK 74137

Oregon

PMS Treatment Center   (503) 255-0918
10373 N.E. Hancock   Phil Alberts, M.D., F.A.C.O.G.
P.O. Box 20998   Suzanne L. Alberts, R.N.C.
Portland, OR 97220-0998   Michael S. Alberts, Ph.D.

Pennsylvania

Matrix PMS Clinic   (412) 782-2992/4700
135 Freeport Road   Christiane M. F. Siewers, M.D.
Pittsburgh, PA 15215   Mary Kay Lewis

U. of Pennsylvania PMS Program   (215) 662-3329
Deptartment of Ob/Gyn   Steven J. Sondheimer, M.D.
U. of Pennsylvania Hospital   Ellen W. Freeman, Ph.D.
3400 Spruce Street
Philadelphia, PA 19104

Tennessee

Vanderbilt University PMS Program (615) 322-6576
Center for Fertility & Reproductive Research
Vanderbilt U. Medical Center North, Rm. D-3223
Nashville, TN 37232 Joel Hargrove, M.D.

Texas

PMS Center of Irving Texas (214) 579-0551
1430 MacArthur, Ste. 103 Frank Knopp, M.D.
Irving, TX 75061

PMS Medical Clinic (214) 368-4457
7424 Greenville Avenue, Ste. 205 Lorayne Genaro, M.D.
Dallas, TX 75231 Peter Boger, M.A.

Utah

Deborah F. Robinson, M.D. (801) 533-8030
324 10th Avenue, Ste. 154 Deborah F. Robinson, M.D.
Salt Lake City, UT 84103

PMS Specialists of Utah (801) 584-2105
501 Chipeta Way, Ste. 1250 Richard Shanteau, M.D.
Salt Lake City, UT 84108 Leanne Geigle

Wisconsin

Eau Claire Clinic, Ltd. (715) 834-3171
2103 Heights Drive, Box 264 Albert A. Lorenz, M.D.
Eau Claire, WI 54702 Sharon A. Heinz, M.S.E.

GROUPS WITH NO MEDICAL DIRECTOR

California

* Parenting Center (213) 476-8561, ext. 209
Stephen S. Wise Temple Marilyn Brown, Director
15500 Stephen S. Wise Drive Norma Freeman
Los Angeles, CA 90077

Channel Island Center For Women's Health   (805) 656-3310
3160 Loma Vista, Ste. B   Mary Jones,R.N.,M.N.
Ventura, CA 93003   Debby Haberthur

† PMS Center of California   (209) 956-4767
615 Lincoln Center   Marcia Fry-Galbraith, Director
Stockton, CA 95207   Michelle Tuitavuki

PMS Relief, Inc.   (916) 888-7677
11710 Education Street   Gillian Ford
Auburn, CA 95603-2499   Katie Lynch

Illinois

* PMS Center Of Illinois   (708) 520-3822
942 Twisted Oak Lane   Linaya Hahn Back
Buffalo Grove, IL 60089

Indiana

PMS Community Awareness   (812) 372-5340
1914 Chandler Lane   Laurie Woodall
Columbus, IN 47203

Massachusetts

* Northshore Women's Care   (617) 942-0743
511 Pearl Street   Laurea Nugent, R.N.C.
Reading, MA 01867

Minnesota

PMS Discovery, Support & Training Center   (612) 472-5311
5023 Edgewater Drive   Joy Bennet
Mound, MN 55364

PMS Clinic of Minneapolis, Inc.   (612) 830-0990
200 Edina Professional Building   Jane A. Trimble, M.S., R.N.
7250 France Ave. South
Minneapolis, MN 55435

Montana

Blue Mountain Women's Clinic
715 Kensington, Ste. 24
Missoula, MT 59801

(406) 721-1646
Tracy Mikkola, Director
Louise Flanagan, R.N.

Nevada

PMS Research Foundation
P.O. Box 14574
Las Vegas, NV 89114

(702) 369-9248
Lee Horner

New York

Nassau County Office of Women's Services
243 Fulton Avenue
Hempstead, NY 11550

(516) 564-8250
Geraldine Linton
Joan Olbergh

Ohio

Guidance Center of Ashland
PumpHouse Square
400 Orange Street, Ste. 300
Ashland, OH 44805

(419) 289-2522
Roger D. Osborn, Ph.D.
N. Ruth Mistie, A.C.S.W.

Oklahoma

University Of Oklahoma
College of Medicine, Dept. of Ob/Gyn
P.O. Box 26901, 4SP Room 503
Oklahoma City, OK 73190

(405) 271-8719
Jody Boren, M.S.W.

Oregon

Robert Sklovsky, Naturopathic Physician
10808 S.E. Highway 212
Clackamas, OR 97015

(503) 656-0707
Robert Sklovsky, Pharm. D., N.D.

Texas

Ray's Pharmacy, Inc.
400 S. Main
Mansfield, TX 76063

(800) 255-7135
Danny Ray, R.Ph.
Gary Wynn, R.Ph.

Prof. Compounding Centers of America   (800) 331-2498
10925 Kinghurst, Ste. 520   David Sparks, R.Ph.
Houston, TX 77099   George Webber

Wisconsin

Metabolic Analysis Labs, Inc.   (608) 255-2491
1202 Ann Street   A.L. Shug, Ph.D.
Madison, WI 53713   K. J. Shug

* PMS Access   (800) 222-4PMS
Madison Pharmacy Assciates   in WI: (608) 833-4PMS
P.O. Box 9326   Marla Ahlgrimm, R.Ph.
Madison, WI 53715   David Myers, R.Ph.

Women's International Pharmacy   (800) 234-0458
9500 Monona Drive   Wallace L. Simons, R.Ph.
P.O. Box 6468
Madison, WI 53716–0468

INDEX

———————— 🙟 ————————

Absenteeism 115–116
Accidents 116
Acne 64, 69, 155
Adolescence 81–89
Adrenalin 150–151
Alcohol, sensitivity to, 3, 23, 34, 61, 62, 71, 98, 105, 126, 191
Alcoholism, 132
Amenorrhea (absence of menstruation) 31, 32, 121–122, 133, 158–160
Amnesia 132
Anemia 163
Anorexia nervosa 31, 85, 137, 160
Anovular cycle 98, 170
Anxiety 17, 151
Arthritis, rheumatoid, 18
Aspirin 58
Asthma 1, 2, 6, 17, 23, 52, 63–65, 115
Athletes and PMS, 121–123

🙟 ——————————

Backache 17, 24, 51
Biorhythms 135
Birth control (see contraception; pill, contraceptive)
Bladder infections 64
Bloatedness 24, 47–53, 64
Blood pressure 32, 48, 200
Blood sugar level and PMS xiii, 34–35, 44, 53, 59–61, 98, 104, 109, 149–152, 189
Boils 69

Bones 122, 167, 172, 180, 192
Breast soreness 49–50, 64
Breastfeeding 159
Breasts 81, 146, 195
Bromocriptine 50, 97, 167, 212
Bronchitis 18

🙟 ——————————

Caffeine 192
Calcium 122, 167, 172, 193
Cancer 195, 199–201, 208
Candida (yeast) 208
Cannabis 126
Carbohydrates 149, 190
Carpal tunnel syndrome 52
Cervix 161
Chart, menstrual 24–30
Cheese 61, 62
Child abuse 3, 45, 112–113
Children and PMS 107–114
Chocolate 61, 62
Cholesterol 170
Citrus fruits, 61, 62
Clinics, PMS, 220–221, 235–244
Clonidine 214–215
Conception 211
Congestive dysmenorrhea 74, 77–78
Conjunctivitis, 70, 146
Conn's syndrome 53
Constipation 191
Contact lenses 23, 50, 71
Contraception 109–110, 163, 210–211
Coronary disease 170, 172, 200
Cortisone 172

Crime and PMS, 45–46, 28–134
Cyclical idiopathic edema 49
Cystitis 64, 69

❧ ————————

Dalton Society, 220
Decongestants 57
DES (stilbestrol) 195, 208
Depression 17, 35, 37–40, 51,
    64, 86, 97, 137, 166–167
Depressive illness 160
Diet 189–192, 203
Dieting 53, 85, 160
Dihydrotestosterone 145
Dilatation and curettage
    (D&C) 75
Dioenestrol 195
Diuretics 52–53, 215
Dizziness 50
Driving 123–124
Drug reactions 71
Drug treatments
    bromocriptine 50, 97, 167, 212
    clonidine 214–215
    diuretics 52–53, 215
    estrogen therapy 195–199
    potassium 47, 52, 53, 215
    progesterone therapy 1, 53,
        54, 58, 87, 98, 105, 202–208
    prostaglandin inhibitors 77,
        84, 187, 195
    pyridoxine (Vitamin B-6)
        212–214
Dysmenorrhea 74–80
    congestive 74, 77–78
    spasmodic 32, 84, 74–77, 91,
        115, 155–156, 167, 173,
        186–187, 195–196

❧ ————————

Edema 49
"Empty nest" syndrome 183–184

Endometriosis 78–80
Epilepsy 1, 3, 17, 19, 64, 65–66,
    151
Estrogen 10, 12, 17, 69, 77, 84,
    119, 122, 140, 181
Estrogen deficiency 157–158,
    173–174
Estrogen implants 164, 198
Estrogen therapy 194–199
Eyes
    conjunctivitis 70, 146
    contact lenses 23, 50, 71
    glaucoma 18, 52, 70, 146
    iritis 70
    pressure, 48, 50
    sties, 69, 146
    uveitis 70, 146

❧ ————————

Fainting 69
Fatigue 17, 35, 40–43
"Feedback pathway," hormonal
    141
Fertilization 10
Fibroids, 161, 163
Follicle Stimulating Hormone
    (FSH) 17, 139, 163
Follicle Stimulating Hormone
    Releasing Hormone
    (FSHRH) 139
Food cravings 70–71

❧ ————————

Gambling 126
Glaucoma 18, 52, 70, 146
Glucocorticoid receptors 154
Graafian follicle 10

❧ ————————

Hay fever 68, 146
Headaches 17, 18, 24, 50, 52,
    54–62, 64

migraine 1–12, 52, 54, 55, 57, 58–62, 64, 115, 151, 165
sinus (vacuum) 51, 56–58
tension 57, 58
Heart disease 170, 172, 200
Herpes 110
Hexoestradiol 195
Homicide 16, 45
Hormone blood tests 29–30
Hormone receptors 146
Hormone Replacement Treatment 174
Hormone variations, male and female (chart) 13
Hormones
corticosteroids 172
estrogen 10, 12, 17, 69, 77, 84, 119, 122, 140, 181
Follicle Stimulating Hormone (FSH) 17, 139, 163
Follicle Stimulating Hormone Releasing Hormone (FSHRH) 139
Luteinising hormone (LH) 17, 139, 140, 163
Luteinising hormone releasing hormone (LHRH) 139
progesterone xiii, 10, 17, 29, 32, 78, 110, 140, 146–149, 219
prolactin 50, 141
prostaglandin 77, 155
Sex Hormone Binding Globulin (SHBG) xii, 29, 145–146
testosterone 168, 172, 211–212
Hot flashes 177–178
Human chorionic gonadotrophin 159
Husband battering 45, 96
Husbands and PMS, 1, 2, 4, 11, 43, 90–99, 100–106
Hyperglycemia 149

Hypoglycemia 149, 152
Hypothalamus 137, 138, 139, 144
Hysterectomy 162–168, 172

❧ ——————

Ibuprofen (Advil, Motrin, Nuprin) 195
Implants
estrogen 164–198
progesterone 206–207
testosterone 211–212
Indomethacin (Indocin) 195
Infanticide 16, 133
Insulin 149
Iritis 70
Irregular menstruation 83–84
Irritability 17, 24, 43–46, 151

❧ ——————

Karyopicnotic Index 182

❧ ——————

Lamb, Charles and Mary 101–102
Laparscopy 79
Laryngitis 146
Lesbians 145
Luteinising hormone (LH) 17, 139, 140, 163
Luteinising hormone releasing hormone (LHRH) 139

❧ ——————

"Male menopause" 183
Magnesium 214
Marriage and PMS 2–4, 90–99, 167
Mastitis 146
Mefanamic acid (Ponstel) 195
Men and PMS, 1, 2, 4, 11, 43, 90–99, 100–106
Menarche 81–83, 174
Menopausal flushes 177–178

Menopause 20, 85, 158, 164, 169–184
  age at 174–175
  hormonal changes 170–173
  symptoms of 177–182
  treatment of 192–193
Menstrual chart 24–30, 103
Menstrual clock 139–141, 159
Menstrual controlling center 137–139
Menstrual cycle 10–11, 12–14, 135–152
  variation in length of, 11–12, 136–137
Menstrual distress, definition 17
Menstrual synchrony 95, 114, 144–145
Menstruation
  attitudes toward 14–15
  description of, 6, 10
  effect of emotions on, 143–144
  myths and customs 8–10, 81–82
"Mid-thirties" syndrome 20
Migraine headaches 1–12, 52, 54, 55, 57, 58–62, 64, 115, 151, 165
  and blood sugar level 59–61
  and diet 61–62
  classical 58
  common 58
  trigger factor 59
Mittelschmerz (ovulation) 72
Mood swings 16, 20, 85, 182
Moos Menstrual Distress Questionnaire 23
Mothers and PMS 107–114
Multiple sclerosis 18
Murder 16, 45

ᴥ ─────────

Naproxen (Naprosyn) 195
National PMS Society 216–217

Nutrition and PMS 189–192
Nymphomania 132

ᴥ ─────────

Oophorectomy (removal of ovaries) 162–168
Osteoporosis 122, 167, 172, 180, 192
Ovaries 10, 139, 162–168
Ovulation 10, 14, 72, 74, 84, 97–98, 139, 140, 141–143, 160, 167
  determining timing of 141–143

ᴥ ─────────

Pain, menstrual (*see also* dysmenorrhea) 5, 32, 78–80
Panic attacks 151
Paracetamol 58
Phenylethylamine 61
Pheromones 145
Phosphorus 172
Pill, contraceptive 31, 32–33, 55, 75, 84, 97, 110, 123, 133, 136, 158
Pituitary gland 141
Polyps 161
Postnatal depression 32, 65, 133
Potassium 47, 52, 53, 215
Pre-eclamptic toxemia 32, 65, 133
Pregnancy 31, 32, 55, 74, 75, 92, 97, 133, 148, 158, 210
Pregnancy tests 158–159
Premenstrual syndrome and
  accidents 116
  adolescence 27, 31–32
  alcohol 3, 23, 34, 61, 62, 71, 98, 105, 126, 191
  child abuse 3, 45, 112–113
  crime 45–46, 128–134
  drug reactions 71
  exercise 121–123, 186–187

hospitalization 116
hysterectomy 165
medical profession 9, 21–22, 217–218
men 1, 2, 4, 11, 43, 90–99, 100–106
pill, contraceptive 31, 32–33, 55, 75, 84, 97, 110, 123, 133, 136, 158
pregnancy 108
puberty 31, 81–83, 133, 140
stress 159
suicide 3, 16, 38–39, 86
tension 17, 18, 35–47
Premenstrual syndrome, causes 153–161
Premenstrual syndrome, definition 16, 17
Premenstrual syndrome, diagnosis of 21–34, 131–134
Premenstrual syndrome, effect on driving 123–124
hobbies 123
marriage 2–4, 90–99, 167
schoolwork 42–43, 87–89, 144
sense of smell 68
sexual desire 86, 104, 133, 176, 183
shopping 124–125
sports 121–123
vacation 126–127
work 115–120
Premenstrual syndrome, symptoms 63–72, 153–154
asthma 1, 2, 6, 17, 23, 52, 63–65, 115
bloatedness 24, 47–53, 64
breast soreness 49–50, 64
conjunctivitis 70, 140
cystitis 64, 69
depression 17, 35, 37–40, 51, 64, 86, 97, 137, 166–167

dizziness 50
epilepsy 1, 3, 17, 19, 64, 65–66, 151
eye pressure 48
fainting 69
fatigue 17, 35, 40–43
food cravings 70–71
glaucoma 18, 52, 70, 146
headaches 17, 18, 24, 50, 52, 54–62, 64
irritability 17, 24, 43–46, 151
joint and muscle pains 69
laryngitis 146
mood swings 16–20, 85
personality changes 6
rhinitis (hayfever) 68, 146
sinusitis 146
ulcers 71
urethritis 69
varicose veins 69
vertigo 68
water retention 47–53
weight gain 17, 18, 32, 47, 48, 139, 167
Premenstrual syndrome, treatment medical 194–215
self 185–193
Premenstrual tension (PMT) 35–47
Progesterone xiii, 10, 17, 29, 32, 78, 110, 140, 146–149, 219
Progesterone deficiency 157, 163, 172–173
Progesterone implants 206–207
Progesterone receptors 147–149, 154
Progesterone therapy 1, 53, 54, 58, 87, 98, 105, 202–208
Progestogens 29, 201, 208–210
Prolactin 50, 141
Prostaglandin 77, 155
Prostaglandin inhibitors 77, 84, 187, 195

Puberty 31, 81–83, 133, 140
Pyridoxine (Vitamin B-6) 50, 191–192, 212–214

❧ ⸺⸺⸺⸺⸺

Receptors
    glucocorticoid 154
    progesterone 147–149, 154
Relaxation exercises 186–187
Rheumatic pain 51
Rhinitis (hayfever) 68, 146

❧ ⸺⸺⸺⸺⸺

Schizophrenia 18
School and PMS 42–43, 87–89, 144
Self-mutilation 39–40
Sex Hormone Binding Globulin (SHBG) xiii, 29, 145–146
Sexual activity and PMS 86, 104, 133, 176, 183
Shoplifting 3, 23, 125, 129
Sinusitis 17
Skin and PMS 64, 69, 155
Skin lesions 64
Smoking 77, 175, 192
    effect on age at menopause 175, 192
Spasmodic dysmenorrhea 32, 84, 74–77, 91, 115, 155–156, 167, 173, 186–187, 195–196
Sports 121–123
Sterilization 65, 133, 163, 211
Stilbestrol (DES) 195, 208
Stress 159
Suicide 3, 16, 38–39, 86
Suppositories, progesterone 204–205

Tamoxifen 199–200
Tension 17, 18, 35–47
Tereshkova, Valentina (Soviet cosmonaut) 118
Testosterone 168, 172, 211–212
Testosterone implants 212
Tubal ligation 33, 110
Tyramine 61, 62

❧ ⸺⸺⸺⸺⸺

Ulcers 71
University of Oklahoma, Department of Premenstrual Syndrome 218
Urethritis 64
Uterus 162, 163
Uveitis 70

❧ ⸺⸺⸺⸺⸺

Vasodilating amines 61
Vertigo 64
Victoria (Queen of England) 3–4, 101
Vitamin B-6 (pyridoxine) 50, 191–192, 212–214

❧ ⸺⸺⸺⸺⸺

Water retention 47–52
Weight-gain 17, 18, 32, 47, 48, 139, 167
Weight swings 33, 139, 159

❧ ⸺⸺⸺⸺⸺

Yeast infections (Candida) 20

MENOPAUSE WITHOUT MEDICINE
by Linda Ojeda, Ph.D.

Having researched and studied menopause for many years, Linda Ojeda has written a current and complete handbook for the woman interested in caring for herself and preparing for the change.

Part One explains the causes of common menopausal symptoms—insomnia, hot flashes, fatigue, osteoporosis—and natural ways to treat them.

Part Two is about aging gracefully. Your personal appearance, sexuality, and energy level can have a strong impact on your overall well-being.

Part Three emphasizes good lifestyle habits, which can make the difference between a carefree menopause and a difficult one.

This important book is for the aware woman who wants the best out of life at every age.

Soft Cover ... 288 pages ... $11.95

THE ENABLER: When Helping Harms the Ones You Love
by Angelyn Miller

The concept of enabling or co-dependency is well known to addiction counselors, as well as to members of Al-Anon, CoA, and other groups for families of addicts. Yet thousands of people who do not have a problem with chemical dependency enable their spouses, children, and friends without ever realizing that their helpfulness harms the people they love.

Angelyn Miller describes how she came to the painful realization that she was an enabler, even though there was no history of alcoholism or drug addiction in her family. She offers a way out, sharing insights, and giving specific techniques and tools for transforming dysfunctional relationships into healthy ones. In going beyond the addiction recovery audience, THE ENABLER continues and strengthens the work begun in Melody Beattie's *Co-dependent No More.*

Soft Cover ... 144 pages ... $6.95

To order, please see last page

ORDER FORM

NAME

ADDRESS

CITY   STATE

ZIP   COUNTRY

TITLE	QTY	PRICE	TOTAL
The Enabler		@ $ 6.95	
Exclusively Female		@ $ 5.95	
Getting High in Natural Ways		@ $ 6.95	
Healthy Aging *(paperback)*		@ $ 11.95	
Healthy Aging *(hard cover)*		@ $ 17.95	
Helping Your Child Succeed After Divorce		@ $ 9.95	
Lupus: My Search for a Diagnosis		@ $ 6.95	
Menopause Without Medicine		@ $ 11.95	
Once A Month *4th Edition*		@ $ 9.95	
PMS: Premenstrual Syndrome		@ $ 6.95	
Self-Help for PMS		@ $ 9.95	
Sexual Healing		@ $ 12.95	

Shipping costs:
First book: $2.00
($3.00 for Canada)
Each additional book:
$.50 ($1.00 for Canada)
For UPS rates and bulk orders call us at (714) 624-2277

TOTAL
Less discount @_____%   (   )
TOTAL COST OF BOOKS
Calif. residents add sales tax
Shipping & handling
TOTAL ENCLOSED
Please pay in U.S. funds only

❑ Check   ❑ Money Order   ❑ Visa   ❑ M/C

Card # _____ Exp date _____

Signature _____

Complete and mail to:
Hunter House Inc., Publishers
PO Box 847, Claremont, CA 91711
❑ Check here to receive our book catalog